I0441013

Do These Things or You Will Die
5 Secrets to a Long, Healthy, & Energetic Life!

by

Scott duPont

Contributing author

Ronald Farnham

First Edition

This book is to be read by any person of any age and at any level of health or sickness with results of improved health, vitality, and increased energy. Just like life the more you put into it, the more you will get out of it. Hope you enjoy!

**Do These Things or You Will Die...
5 Secrets to a Long, Healthy & Energetic Life!**

Released and Published by:

Nemours Publishing
c/o Nemours Marketing, Inc.
7531 Azurebrook Court
Winter Park, FL 32792
Tel: (407) 738 – 1608

Do These Things or You Will Die...
5 Secrets to a Long, Healthy & Energetic Life!

ISBN # 9 781481 178655

| U.S. | $9.99 |
| Canada | $12.99 |

Other Books (& Films) by Scott duPont

The ABC's of ACTING (Producer)

ACTING 101 (Producer)

The Greatest Book of Inspiring Quotes (Author)

The BROS. (Producer)

A Dog's Life...The Oscar Lose Story (Executive Producer)

Guerilla Networking (Contributing Author)

MORE Women on Men (Producer)

Sing Along with Holiday Classics (Producer)

What is the Electric Car? (Author)

What is the Electric Car? (Producer)

Who Stole the Electric Car? (Executive Producer)

Women on Men (Producer)

TABLE OF CONTENTS:

SECTION V:
FAITH

Legal Disclaimer:

The title "**Do These Things or You Will Die**" was chosen to grab your attention. There is NO guarantee or implication that the detailed information in this book will help you live forever as everyone will die at some point in their lives, but it is the author's firm belief, however, that understanding the five (5) principles and by implementing the specific and detailed instructions (including the hints, exercises & strategies) in this book will help you live a longer, healthier, and more energetic life!

This book is NOT intended to replace any medical advice or supersede your doctor's specific instructions. This includes instructions to take prescriptions drugs or undergo a life saving surgical procedure. While most of the people we've worked with have gotten off of their prescriptions and medications, they worked closely with their doctors to wean off their medications only after they started showing clear improvements to their health.

This book is NOT an expose about doctors, the medical field, or the pharmaceutical industry, as they all have their proper place. Rather this book will introduce many ideas based upon the long-standing doctrine "Prevention is the best medicine". **It is recommended that ANY alteration of your prescription drug regimen, or the implementation of any exercise program be done with the consultation of a licensed medical, nutritional, or exercise professional.**

In conclusion: NOT "Doing These Things" will most likely decrease your lifespan, and negatively affect your health, your energy, and vitality. If after reading the book, there is any doubt that the information contained in this book did NOT help you become more healthy, simply send back the book for a full refund under Nemours Marketing's 100% Total Satisfaction Guarantee as spelled out at the end of this book.

Author's Qualifications: Why Read this Book?

Because I (the author)…

1) worked for Medco (one of the largest pharmacy benefits management companies in the U.S.) for 8 years. I was on the front lines giving presentations to large employee groups & government agencies as well as fielding questions from employees about their retail & mail-order prescription plans. During that time I spoke to over 12,000 individuals about their prescription medications & ailments.

2) was hired by over a dozen medical equipment & pharmaceutical companies (including Medtronic, Pfizer, Sanofi-Aventis, Merck, Glaxo, Novartis) attending over 100 medical conventions around the world including numerous Oncology annual meetings.

3) worked on a over a dozen medical TV shows including: "Grey's Anatomy", "Private Practice", "Dr. G. Medical Examiner", "Monday Mornings", & "Three Rivers" to name a few and have gotten to learn from the medical technical advisors, writers, and researchers on those sets.

4) although I'm NOT a doctor (I have a great interest in medicine starting when I was "pre-med" in college) and have a ½ dozen family members including cousins who are (or were) M.D.s, PhDs, surgeons, etc. I also read more than 100 books on health, nutrition, and fitness over the past 3 years.

5) have proven LONG TERM RESULTS! Our company has worked with over 50 people (who in as little as 7 days to 3 months) have made dramatic improvements in their health, energy levels and how they feel.

6) am in GREAT health. After changing my diet & exercise regimen over 15 years ago, America's Health Network invited me on their show as their

lowest "Fitness Age®" after multiple of batteries of tests. My Fitness Age® was 16 years younger than my physical age! I say that not to impress you, but to impress upon you that the specific, detailed tools in this book DELIVER RESULTS!

7) I myself (and our research staff at Nemours Marketing) have NO financial ties to any medical institutions, pharmaceutical companies, supplement companies, nutritionists, doctors, or consultants, thus eliminating any possible conflict of interest. I also no longer work for Medco.

8) Read over 100 books on health, diet, nutrition, and exercise as well as dozens of articles on the subjects relevant to assembling this book.

9) lost over a dozen close friends and family members the last few years to cancer and other terminal diseases. My mother and father have fortunately survived cancer, but it is a travesty to lose a stepfather, stepbrother, aunts, uncles, and cousins many of whom were in the prime of their lives. The most shocking losses were my best friend in elementary school (Fritz Collister), my college roommate & fraternity brother (John Clark), and my dear friend and mentor in the film business (Craig Soldinger). Some of these people died in their 30s and 40s! Contributing author Ronald Farnham lost his father to cancer as well which was a driving motivation for him to be involved with this project the past few years. It is my deepest hope that the detailed information in this book will radically improve your health (or simply allow you to maintain your excellent health for the rest of your life) and the life of your loved ones you share this book with as well.

Acknowledgements:

The first time I learned how vitally important Alkalinity is to excellent health was through my friend Tony Robbins. Tony, through all of your detailed research and interviews with world-renowned doctors and experts of this subject, you really enlightened me. You lit a fire in me to research the power of alkalinity even more and I started to share this with as many people as possible. Thank you Tony as well for your research and exploration on the importance of oxygenating cells to preventing cancer and illness. You are one of the most altruistic people I've ever met and I applaud all the lives you have touched and changed for the better.

Thank you also to the dozens of people who trusted me to go through the "7-Day Alkalize & Energize" cleanse program and sharing your amazing results. Special thanks to my lifelong friend Bill Hartranft and the commitment you made to lose the weight and take back your health.

To Bruce Ellington, thank you for all your feedback, support, notes, etc. while "on set". I should probably thank your superstar wife Jill as well, for inspiring us both to be as healthy as we can be and avoiding so many of today's foods that have become poisonous and toxic. I hope that your dad reads this book so that you and your family can all share his 100th birthday together in the future.

To Desmond Bailey, despite being such a skeptic at the beginning, I appreciate your trust in me and for following the program. I'm thrilled that you had such great results. I hope that you share the book with your loved ones that you care about.

Thanks to Aleksandra Kyoseva for being the very first interview for the documentary film version of this book. I appreciate your candidness about your sickness created by the new American diet having moved here just a few years ago from rural Romania.
Thank you as well to my research team at Nemours Marketing, Inc. including Scott Townsend. Even your work part-time has been a huge help with this project.

To Ronald Farnham, thanks for your help the past 2 years being involved with this project on a "personal" level and congratulations on claiming your health back and your new healthy lifestyle! I appreciate your being a contributing writer and your help getting this book to press.

Thanks to Andrew Reilly and Nathan Agin on the filming and editing of the IndieGoGo video.

Thank you Dr. Lose for being an inspiration and being one of the many people I know who doesn't pay attention to age. What you've accomplished so far in your life is incredible, and I expect a lot more from you the next 20 - 30 years. I enjoyed our interviews over the phone and hope to see you soon.

To the numerous Medco customers over the last 8 years who volunteered your incredible stories about how you (or your family members) got off of prescriptions, beat cancer and cured yourselves! These inspirational tales clearly demonstrated to me that alternative, holistic therapies are not just for "quacks", but really work!

To my publicist Bill Hooey, thanks in advance for helping spread the word about this book. Whether the book's message helps hundreds, or hundreds of thousands regain their excellent health, I know it can be done with your help in getting this important information out.

Thanks always to my trusted legal council Nicole Weaver. You are truly a "Legal Eagle" with all the help and excellent advice you have provided over the years.

To Monroe Mann for letting me be a contributing writer on your # 1 Best selling book: Guerilla Networking. Your energy, enthusiasm, and passion somehow rubbed off on me and inspired me to write this book to help educate millions of people who need this information!

To Charlotte Gerson, you are my hero for carrying on the life-saving work your father started. I hope to interview you in the near future for the film so we can expand on the plethora of information you share in your great books. What an incredible thing you (and your whole staff) are doing to educate people about the TRUTH about cancer. I applaud you for the countless number of lives you have saved!

Thank you Dr. Robert Young and Shelley Young. Your many years of research and work specifically into alkalizing our bodies and through your renowned book series The pH Miracle, has saved thousands of lives. Keep up the great work!

Thanks lastly to Jaime Oliver and Ryan Seacrest. Your passion in starting at the grassroots level with the inner cities and in the schools, etc. is to be applauded. You have targeted ground zero where obesity is at its worst and educating and inspiring all walks of life and all ages to re-gain their health.

Dedication:

This book is dedicated to all my family members still alive including my **Mom**. Life is short and it is my sincere hope that by applying the specific strategies and tools in this book, you may all live a long, healthy, and energetic life so we can enjoy and celebrate many more good times together.

To my many fallen family members and close friends including Phi Delta Theta "Brother" **John Clark** who left way too early, I think of you often and hope this book makes a difference in saving many lives.

"If I'd known I was going to live so long,
I'd have taken better care of myself."
- Leon Eldred

Forward:

As mentioned, I lost several family members and close friends the past few years including many who died far too young. Even though I lost touch with John Clark the last few years, I was absolutely shocked when my former roommate and fraternity brother died of cancer. Then when cancer took away my mentor and close friend Craig Soldinger, that was devastating. Simultaneously while these family members and close friends passed away, I was making some disturbing observations working for Medco. I was hired during the "open enrollment" period in the fall when large businesses, schools, and government agencies would host health benefit fairs to educate their employees about their health insurance options for the upcoming year. I would make presentations to all the employees about changes in their prescription benefits plan and later would staff the Medco table where people would come by for one-on-one questions. The questions were normally about when a generic drug would become available (which would save them a LOT of money) and then if someone were at the point where they were taking a "maintenance" medication (such as a high blood pressure drug, a cholesterol prescription, etc.), I would educate them about how to enroll in a mail-order plan where they could get a 90-day supply for a substantial discount vs. the typical 30-day supply at the retail pharmacy. People now could get 3 times as many pills shipped directly to their home for a discount. In the 8 years I worked for Medco, the people who signed up for the mail order (who were stuck taking maintenance prescriptions on a regular basis), were normally people in their 50s or 60s, and sometimes retirees who were even older. This last year I worked these benefit fairs for Medco (all over the country), I was absolutely shocked to see more and more people in their 20s or 30s who were hooked on blood pressure statins or cholesterol medications in addition to their ADHD medications! Some of theses employees (less than 30 years old) were already taking 2 – 3 different prescription regimens on a daily basis and did not represent the health and vitality I had seen in the younger employees just a few years earlier. Over the past 2 years, I saw a noticeable rise in employees battling cancer or the lucky ones who were recovering from a long, harsh battle with cancer treatments. While I can't tell you the exact count, I saw over 12,000 employees on a one-on-one basis who came to the table to speak with me, and I would estimate in the last 2 years of benefit fairs I worked, the number of people I spoke to who told me about their cancer was up at least 300% (3 times higher) than just a few years prior. It's no secret anymore that a health epidemic is coming. The World Health Organization stated that 41% of Americans will be diagnosed with cancer in their lifetimes! Statistics from the American Heart Association show that 75 million Americans currently suffer from heart disease, 20 million have diabetes and 57 million have pre-diabetes. Millions of kids and teenagers now have diabetes for the very first time! These disorders are affecting younger people in greater numbers every year as the obesity rate continues to skyrocket. At the same time, two of the many people we've interviewed so far for the documentary film version of this book (Crystal Wei from China and Aleksandra Kyoseva from Romania) both told us in their interviews that neither of them had a single family member who had even been diagnosed with cancer! This is not to say that cancer and other terminal illnesses do not exist in these countries, but prior to both of these ladies moving to the United States, they both bicycled to school, ate fresh vegetables from their own gardens, led very active and healthy lifestyles compared to their American counterparts. Of course when they moved to the U.S. in the mid to late 90s, fast foods, sodas, energy drinks, and "flavored" water had not yet saturated their countries.

There are dozens of statistics (and quite frankly horrific trends) the CDC and Stand Up 2 Cancer [F-1] have been tracking the last few years including:

1) **Infertility** in this country. What used to be a rarity (fecundity – the impaired ability for women to have children) now affects 6.9 million women ages 15 - 44 each year!

2) The U.S. claims top honors in the world for **bone degeneration** with almost 10% of Americans estimated to suffer from osteoporosis. The estimated figure is between 28 and 30 million people in this country, so how is that native people living traditional lifestyles around the world have been classified as "almost immune" to osteoporosis by doctors in Asia and Africa?

3) **Obesity** is even hitting the U.S. Army, which kicked out 1,625 soldiers for being out of shape so far this year. That's 15 times the number discharged in 2007! [F-2]

4) Just a few decades ago, most Americans didn't even know what the word **Autism** was let alone know anybody who had an autistic kid. The incidence in children in 1970 was just 1 in 10,000. The March CDC 2012 reports show that 1 out of 88 children are now affected with autism!

Now before I get sidetracked with dozens more statistics and stories on how abysmal the results for the U.S. health care system is, let's get back to the story. My mother & father have fortunately survived cancer, but it is a travesty to lose a stepfather, stepbrother, aunts, uncles, and cousins, many of whom were not that old. The most shocking losses were my best friend in elementary school Fritz Collister, as mentioned my college roommate & fraternity brother John Clark, and my dear friend and mentor in the film business Craig Soldinger. Some of these people died in their 30s and 40s! Little did I know at the time while I was out educating sick people about prescription drugs, I was also getting an education myself from cancer survivors and motivated individuals who had enough of their obesity, allergies, diabetes, or arthritis and shared their incredible recovery stories with me. Over the last 15 years attending medical conferences (including the annual Clinical Oncology conventions), and then the past 8 years working for Medco very clear trends emerged that MOST of these medical issues including cancer can be avoided! About the same time I was introduced to the powerful concept of "alkalizing" your body from my friend

Tony Robbins (who had done an extraordinary amount of research on the subject), and also got introduced to Dr. Theodore Baroody and his book <u>Alkalize or Die</u>. While I don't want to allude to the readers of this book that alkalizing (or oxygenating – the other KEY factor to excellent health) is a 100% guarantee of perfect health or avoidance of cancer, it is absolutely mind boggling to see the positive results that can be obtained from the specific, preventative measures of diet & exercise I've outlined in the chapters ahead. It is my deepest hope that the detailed information in this book will change your life and the life of your loved ones you choose to share this book with as well. Dr. Max Gerson at one point had a 74% success rate in curing his cancer victims and many of the principles in the "alkaline" section were initially discovered and proven to work by him and now carried on by his daughter Charlotte at The Gerson Clinic. Although all cancers and treatments vary, success at some of the best cancer treatment centers in the world is less 30%! This book is all about quantitative FACTS and PROVEN RESULTS. I hope that upon conclusion of the book, it will have opened your eyes up to a whole new world of possibilities including a long, healthy, & energetic life!

"Health is like money,
we never have a true idea of its value until we lose it."
- Josh Billings

How the Information in this Book
Changed My Life in Just 7 Days!

by contributing author Ronald Farnham

I've known Scott for almost 15 years now after meeting on the set of "Larry the Cable Guy, Health Inspector"...a film we both worked on which shot at Universal Studios Florida. I was in great shape then due to my military background. I had enlisted for 8 years with the U.S. Army, and later served 6 additional years as an independent contractor including military intelligence work in Germany, Mexico, and South Korea. Although I am extremely busy with several other book projects and screenplays I'm writing at the moment, I agreed to help out with the research the past 2 years and write this short chapter because this subject of health is personal to me, as my father died of cancer. Like most people, I also have several family members and close friends who are either obese or suffering some medical ailments. My mother now is showing some ailments, which I'm 100% convinced are a result of an acidic diet. I pray that she reads this book as the concept of alkalinity (which Scott will go into in great detail is absolutely critical to good health). In fact in our research and "informal" polls, we could NOT find a single person who had major health ailments including heart disease, diabetes, high blood pressure, arthritis, osteoporosis, or gout who was a strict vegetarian or someone who had a plant based (80 – 90% "alkaline") diet.

Scott and I always kept in touch and the relevant story here begins 10 years later when he picked me up at LAX airport. I was relocating to Hollywood to work on my own screenplays and develop some new film projects. Scott and I were going to be sharing a small studio space in North Hollywood where Scott had just completed 2 films. Scott hadn't seen me in almost 5 years and admitted later that he didn't recognize me at first when driving along the airport curbside to pick me up. I didn't realize it (perhaps it was denial, perhaps because my lifestyle after the military had changed), but I was more than 60 lbs. overweight and not in the best physical condition. Scott took me on a 5 mile hike in the Hollywood Hills the first weekend I arrived and I was definitely a little winded and sweating quite a bit even though it was neither hot nor humid. I noticed that Scott was a little leaner, didn't look any older, and had more energy than he'd ever had before. He mentioned in passing that he was going to do his annual "7 Day Alkalize + Energize" cleanse. If you look at Scott's library of films and documentaries as well as his newspaper and magazine columns over the years, he has always been interested in educating and enlightening people in a positive way, so I was intrigued when he told me about his new health program enough to give it a try. The word "try" should be a clue that this would not deliver the best results for me. Scott and I both began his special liquid diet for 7 days, which involved juicing fresh alkaline vegetables 2- 3 times a day and drinking lots of alkaline water. Scott was very meticulous in his process including taking "before" and "after" photos of himself, and he asked whoever was in the studio to confirm his or her weight each day (at the same exact time) before he logged that info into a weight tracker spread sheet. Scott also had a journal where he would write copious notes about how he slept each night, how his energy levels were, if he had any energy spikes, noting exactly what he drank, how much, and when, etc. This seemed a little too detailed for me, but I did follow his plan and drank lemon water and vegetable juice every single day and started feeling better after the first day. There were several items I totally disagreed with Scott on including his mandate of not doing any major exercise (especially weight lifting or P-90X strength training that I was doing) during the 7 days of the alkaline cleanse. I thought this was ridiculous for anyone wanting to lose weight. Scott also had this strict rule of no fruits, which included healthy foods I love like bananas, oranges, apples, and avocados. This did not make sense to me either. After doing my own research, I concluded these fruits had alkaline properties and were very healthy, so I chose to sneak in a few pieces of fruit each day in between my juicing. After 7 days, I felt better and had more energy and although I lost a few pounds here and there at the end of 7 days, my net loss was only 1.5 pounds! Scott on the other hand (who was not fat to begin with) lost an average of 2 pounds each day for a net loss of 14.2 pounds and shrunk 2 belt sizes. Also with the massive hydration he gave his body (his diet was only liquids for those 7 days), his skin looked noticeably better.

Hopefully Scott will go into all the technical details of why his 7 days were a success, and although I felt better and lost a few pounds, my results were not what he expected based upon the results of all the other people he had worked with on his 7-day alkaline program. I later admitted to Scott that I had done 2 sessions of P-90X and had snuck in a few pieces of fruit during the 7 days. He was adamant that extreme exercise creates lactic acid and he also mentioned that since fruits are loaded with sugar, that sugar in turn is acidic. While I was still skeptical that such a simple easy program could work, Scott shared some amazing before and after photos of one of his best friends (Bill Hartranft) who lost 41.6 pounds in the first 42 days and was feeling much better by losing that extra weight. I have never been a quitter, so a few weeks later I told Scott I was ready to do the 7 Day "Alkalize + Energize" cleanse exactly the way he suggested. This time I was not going to "cheat", but promised to him (and most importantly to myself) that I would follow the program with military precision. After a large feast that our mutual co-producer friend Andrew cooked for all of us including chicken, salad, pasta, bread, cheese & crackers, and a few glasses of wine, the next morning I was ready for the official weigh in at the studio the next morning. I weighed in at just over 225 pounds, which is heavy for someone under 6 feet tall. I'm sure Scott will detail the step by step process of his "7 Day Alkalize + Energize" program and sticking to his rules, I lost 1 – 2 pounds every single day just like clockwork. While I lost 17 pounds at the end of that first week, the primary thing I noticed was that my energy level was through the roof! Also the vegetable juice, which had tasted very bitter the first few days, started tasting sweet. I also noticed I had absolutely no joint pain in my shoulder which can sometimes be a little sore after a baseball game, as I used to be a professional baseball player and still get paid from time to time to pitch in minor league games. I found I really enjoyed my trips to the grocery store every other day to pick out different raw vegetables and fell in love with the process of juicing where my body got an immediate energy boost from all the liquid nutrients which are rapidly absorbed. Unlike caffeine (I used to be a big coffee drinker), the new energy I got did not seem to fade as long as I was juicing or hydrating every few hours with lemon water. After the 7th day, I chose to continue with the same juicing program, since it was working so well for me and I did not miss the processed, store bought food I had been dumping in my body. The short version of this story is that I continued the program for 90 days. On the 90th day, I met with Scott and one other witness in the studio for the official weigh in. I weighed exactly 165 pounds! The results were a whopping 60-pound weight loss in a relatively short time frame without any extreme exercise. I'm a firm believer that these results were from alkalizing my system and expelling toxins, which had built up over many years in my system. While I tell people that the 60-pound weight loss was a significant milestone (and I gave Scott permission to print the photos taken on Day 1 and Day 90 for this book), the most important benefit to me was my energy level at the end of the 90 days went through the roof. I've always been a night person when writing my screenplays and books, and in the 6 months after cleansing my system, I was writing like a machine until 3 or 4 in the morning. In those 6 months, I finished writing 3 books (all now are published) and completed 4 screenplays, one of which ("Hollywood + Vine") will go into production next month. I also had the energy to write, direct, produce, and edit 20 episodes of my own web series called "The Ronald Show". While I'm proud of these accomplishments this past year, the specific reason I mention this is these creative tasks take a great deal of time and energy and I doubt I would be getting this much work done if I hadn't cleansed my system. I am truly grateful that Scott shared this info with me and turned my health around for the rest of my life. The one note I want to stress is that while the program takes some discipline, it is not hard to complete, and it is not a diet (so you don't go hungry). There is a slight psychological shift in drinking all your meals in a "liquid" (vs. chewing up a big burger or sandwich at each meal), but that did not bother me at all since I felt so good from juicing. The most important thing is to follow his instructions exactly including the "no fruit" and "no solid food" rule for the 7 days. The concept of "Alkalizing" that we've been researching can heal and cure almost any illness or health condition. It is so powerful and I urge you to read that "Alkalize" section carefully and take his 7-day challenge to "Alkalize and Energize"!

The other topics of the book seem overly simplistic, but they really do make sense. When I get in writing mode (just like anyone who works on a computer), I would be seated typing away for 2 – 3 hours at a time and would often get very tired at the end of the day. It does not take a health expert to figure out that a motionless person (unless you want to count my mouse clicks and keyboard strokes as exercise), will get tired after sitting still that long. I've learned never to stay seated at my computer for a period of more than an hour and now break up my writing routine by taking a 5 minute juice break, or go walk around while making a phone call, etc. As simple as it sounds, movement is key to keeping your energy up and staying healthy. In addition to walking (I walk almost every day to the grocery store, or when I am making phone calls, etc.), I now also bike and hike quite often and then a couple times a month will pitch for the local baseball team I'm part of. Tied in with movement and exercise is Scott's concept of "Oxygenating" your body. I now practice deep diaphramic breathing (when walking) and that really helps boost my energy. This is also a worthwhile section of the book to focus on. Once again, it is common sense, but I think in our busy worlds today, we forget to do these things and fall into the trap of being hunched over in front of our computers, breathing shallow breaths for hours at a time. I used to have those bad habits, and just want to know that by setting better habits of excellent posture and doing deep breathing to fully oxygenate your system, you can do wonders for your health and for your energy. The "Hydrate" section of the book is also common sense (my parents always told me to drink more water), but until you instill the habit of drinking 2 – 3 tall glasses of lemon water (which alkalizes your system) each morning, you will not feel the full benefit of hydrating. By drinking lots of alkaline water all day long and snacking on water-rich vegetables and fruits, I no longer get the urge at lunchtime to have a large meal and always have an abundance of energy. Thanks to

Scott, I'm now enjoying perfect health and an abundance of energy I haven't felt since I was a teenager!

"If your body's not right,
the rest of your day will go all wrong.
Take care of yourself."
- **V.L. Allineare**

A SOLUTION to the current health epidemic (the current problems of cancer, disease, and sickness) is this book... **Do These Things or You Will Die** These critical five (5) "Areas" you can master to help live a long, healthy, & energetic life are:

1) ALKALIZE

2) OXYGENATE

3) HYDRATE

4) EXERCISE

5) FAITH

While there's no guarantee you'll cure every illness, disease or beat cancer, in this brand new book, you'll see dozens of examples of people who have gotten healthy, gotten off their medications, and now live their life with a feeling of youth, energy, and vitality. Here's to your own perfect health!

SECTION I:
ALKALIZE

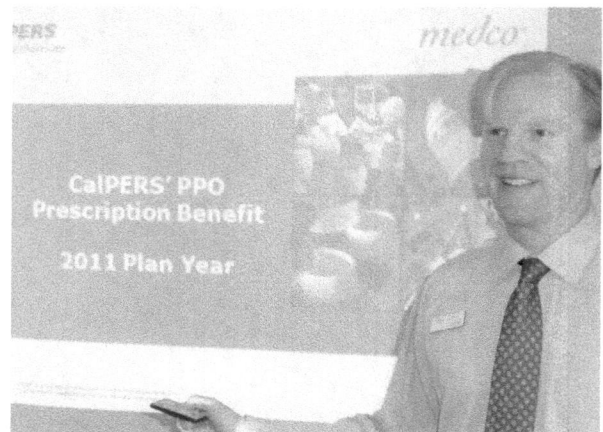

The author Scott duPont hosting a presentation
for Medco at a health benefits fair.

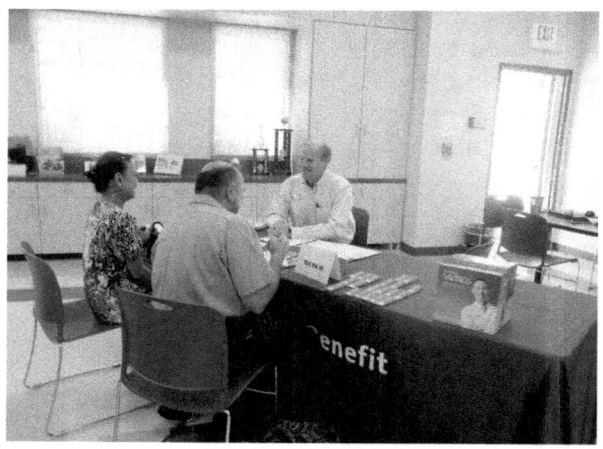

Educating people about maintenance prescriptions
and mail order options.

CHAPTER ONE (1): Don't Take My Word...
<u>Observe the Sick People All Around You!</u>

Alkalizing your body **is by far the MOST important concept and section of this book**. In the next chapter, I'll define the nuts and bolts of alkalinity and the life and death balance of the pH scale. Once you understand the high levels of acidic foods and toxins most of us put in our bodies, you'll be absolutely shocked. The good news is there is an easy fix to turn your body's pH around, and this book will show you a 7-day program that Ronald and I have done many times and that we've shared with dozens of family members and friends that delivers quantitative RESULTS. If you look on the back cover of this book, you'll see some quotes from people who have lost weight, gotten off their prescription drugs, improved their health, and boosted their energy. In this day and age of chronic fatigue (millions of Americans complain about it), who doesn't want more energy? Here are a few notes from the author's journals:

"After I alkalized, I started waking up at 4:30am each morning to write this book and work on other exciting projects. My energy level has gone through the roof and has stayed there ever since." – Scott

"Prior to alkalizing and cleansing my body, I had put on 60 extra lbs. and was very lethargic. I took the 60 lbs. off in just 90 days and now have so much energy that I wrote 3 books and 4 screenplays the last few months, and would rather walk 2 miles to a meeting than get in a car!" – Ronald

Before getting into the specific details of alkalinity, I suggest that you observe and see for yourself the sick people that abound today in the United States. Here are a few eye opening facts:

The U.S. is now the fattest nation among 33 countries with advanced economies, according to a recent report from an international think tank as reported by Nanci Hellmich in USA Today. According to the international study, two-thirds of people in this country are overweight; about a third of adults (more than 72 million) are obese – designated as roughly 30 pounds over a healthy weight. [1-1] At the time of press, nearly half of all adult Americans have high cholesterol, high blood pressure or diabetes according to the CDC. Thomas H. Maugh II of The Los Angeles Times compiled many other staggering statistics in an article appropriately labeled "The Heart Disease Trifecta". [1-2] The prevalence of diabetes is expected to rise sharply over the next 40 years with as many as one in three having the disease. [1-3] The tragic thing of this statistic is that this includes type II diabetes which all medical experts agree in most cases is preventable and even reversible.

Probably the easiest way to measure the sickness of a country is to examine how many people are on prescription drugs. Spending on prescription drugs in the U.S. totaled more than $234.1 billion in 2008, more than double the amount spent in 1999 according to a mind-boggling article in HealthDay about the explosion in prescriptions. [1-4] Recent studies all conclude that prescription drug use in the U.S. continues to rise every single year! It gets much worse when you look at the thousands of prescription drugs that have moved to OTC (over the counter). Most of the statistics and research studies do not factor in the billions of additional pills that people take each day with these drugs.

If these staggering statistics don't prove to you how sick our country is, just take a look the next time you're in line at your local supermarket. Check out the conveyer belt in front of you in line and observe the meats, cheeses, soda, alcohol, chips, dips, ice cream, boxed, frozen, and processed foods that contain tons of sugars and preservatives... all of this is pure acid. Do any of these people look slightly overweight or a little stressed? Now, we know this is very rare, but keep a look out for the person at your local supermarket (or more likely the Whole Foods Market), who sets his or her green vegetables, sprouts, nuts, and fruits on the counter in front of you. Observe carefully and I'm confidant you'll see that these people are usually a lot leaner, have healthier looking skin, and appear more energetic.

Dr. Herbert Ratner who had incredible foresight back in the 1960s said: "Modern man ends up a vitamin-taking, antacid-consuming, barbiturate-sedated, aspirin-alleviated, Benzedrine-stimulated, psychosomatically diseased, surgically despoiled animal; nature's highest product turns out to be a fatigued, peptic-ulcerated, tense, headachy, over-stimulated, neurotic, tonsil-less creature". [1-5] I can only imagine what Dr. Herbert Ratner would say today if he was still alive and saw the amount of Alka-Seltzer, Tums, and antacid prescriptions consumed by a large percentage of the U.S. population.

Here is my frequent observation. I shop at Jon's Market in North Hollywood every 2 – 3 days (as I like my vegetables & fruits fresh), and my abundant supply of colorful, energetic food is usually a huge contrast to the people in front of or behind me in line. Every visit to the grocery store, I'll see a plethora of obese people in line and here is just one example of the person in front of me today: a sickly looking 250 lb. gentleman who was unloading 2 large bottles of Vodka, a 2 liter bottle of Coca-Cola, 2 packages of cured, processed meat (it looked like salami), 1 large package of Kraft cheese slices, 1 pack of cigarettes, 1 large bag of potatoes, 1 really large bag of potato chips, a large package of pita bread, 1 bag of frozen mixed vegetables, and 1 can of sardines. He also had the token name brand 'juice drink', which if you read the fine print on the back of the label is only 15% fruit juice, but mostly comprised of high fructose corn syrup, citric and ascorbic acid, and artificial flavors and coloring. Right before his total was added up, he looked at the counter by the register and grabbed a 5-hour energy drink. I guess with all that crappy, acidic food he was eating for some reason he still needed some energy? I wonder why?

If you're not focused and looking to purchase healthy foods, it can be a challenge in today's grocery stores when so many of the aisles have boxed, bagged, or frozen processed foods many added with preservatives or fillers. Whenever I'm in Florida I usually shop at Publix grocery store. It's interesting that the signs for all the Publix super markets a few years ago used to say: "Publix Market", but their store signs now display: "Publix - Food & Pharmacy". I was told by one source that 80% of the revenues of some grocery stores now comes from their pharmacies and 20% from groceries! I was shocked at first but then realizing that one tiny vial of prescription pills can cost $100, it does not seem so far fetched.

If you still don't think that food trends have drastically changed in grocery stores the past 30 years, don't take my word... do your own observations! Have you ever seen a mother in a supermarket give in to her screaming kid who want a box of Lucky Charms, Sugar Smacks, or Count Chocula cereals? Or do these same mothers get tricked in do buying an Ocean Spray natural Cranberry Drink (on a special sale), which in reality has hardly any cranberry juice in it? Have you ever seen these same parents walk through the freezer section of the grocery store and load up on frozen pepperoni pizzas, or TV dinners with 1 – 2 two token vegetables next to the well-preserved main course meat dish and the sweet sugary dessert. Or perhaps a real treat... some nice steaks on sale for $3.49 per lb. Now that same exact cut of steak labeled truly organic, grass fed, and range-free at the time of publication costs $13.49 per lb. Common sense would tell you that cheap factory meat is not as healthy as organic meat which most people can not afford buying due to the huge cost differential! After the noble gesture of grabbing a few frozen packages of what are labeled as "Healthy" vegetables and perhaps a few token vegetables for a small salad, the hard working mother will cave in to the kids begging for a Twinkie, a few candy bars or perhaps a 5 hour energy drink. More and more kids these days are morbidly obese and many are already taking prescription drugs before they hit their teens! Our research staff found an ABC news report recently, which is quite shocking. It reported an Ohio third-grader who weighed more than 200 pounds that had been taken from his family and placed into foster care after county social workers said his mother wasn't doing enough to control his weight. This poor Cleveland 8-year-old is considered severely obese and at risk for such diseases as diabetes and hypertension. [1-6] I don't know about you, but I never saw a 200 lb. kid in my 3rd grade class! This sad state of affairs is becoming more and more common due to the acidic foods kids are eating and the lack of exercise (which we'll cover in section IV).

I'm not suggesting you have to buy organic foods on your last credit card when you and your family cannot afford it, or that you never ever buy a sweet treat for your kids or yourself after a long day at work. However, I think it's important to really observe how sick, tired, and obese many people in this country are today. If you notice half of the people in your supermarket or even just 30% of the people you see shopping are not healthy... this is the beginning of an epidemic! The good news is you can easily and quickly alkalize your system in just 7 days. But before I explain how to do this, we'll need to define alkalinity and share with you how important this is to you, your family, and your health. I don't want to be all doom and gloom, as there is great news...the next chapter on alkalinity will change your life just like it did for myself (and Ronald) and the dozens of people who we've already shared this information with.

"The appearance of a disease is swift as an arrow; it's disappearance slow, like a thread."
- Chinese Proverb

CHAPTER TWO (2): Definition of ALKALINE

According to the Merriam-Webster dictionary, the definition of ALKALINE is: "of, relating to, containing, or having the properties of an alkali or alkali metal." What you'll find out later is maintaining the properties of your body's alkali metal at the precise level will literally give your body electrical energy just like an alkaline battery does for your flashlight.

Alkaline (or alkalinity) is the opposite of acid (acidic) and is measured with a "basic" pH of slightly above 7 on a scale of 1 to 14. Just as your body functions perfectly at a temperature of 98.6 degrees Fahrenheit, your body (at least your blood stream - also known as the "river of life") functions perfectly at a pH level of 7.36. Throughout this section you'll learn what foods are acidic (examples are coffee, alcohol, meats, most sugar laden foods) and what foods are alkaline (green vegetables, sprouts, almonds, many fruits) and what is the best way to maintain a slightly alkaline environment so that your body functions at its optimal level with much less chance for sickness, disease, and cancer. This section on Alkalinity is the most important concept to understand in the book for your health and for your energy level.

What might be most interesting to you about alkalinity is the energy or "feeling" that the people we've worked with describe how their body felt after a 7-Day "Alkalize & Energize" cleanse. Of course you're more than welcome to extend the program to 10 days, but in just 7 short days, the people you see quoted on the back cover of our book and all the other folks we've helped described their alkaline state with these specific words: "energized", "alive", "super-charged", "vitality", "vigor", "increased stamina", "bouncing off the walls", "excited", "renewed", "rejuvenated", "happy", "healthy" "invincible", "unstoppable" to name a few. Even the most skeptical people previously are not skeptical anymore! Ronald and I get phone calls, e-mails, and letters from new believers every month thanking us for transforming their bodies and boosting their energy levels! Whenever I talk to these people, I also thank them, because they are now spreading the word about how powerful and alkaline diet is and how our 7-Day "Alkalize & Energize" cleanse can and will transform your body (both inside and out). The specifics are laid out in chapter 9, and after you transform your own body and feel the amazing increase in energy, I hope to hear from you as well!

"Our body is a machine for living.
It is organized for that, it is its nature.
Let life go on in it unhindered and let it defend itself,
it will do more than if you paralyze it by encumbering
it with remedies."
- Leo Tolstoy

CHAPTER THREE (3): The History of Food…
<u>How Did it Get So Bad?</u>

I was having an enjoyable, healthy dinner one night with my friends Andrew Reilly and Nathan Agin which lead to some interesting discussions. Nathan is producing a web series for travelers on how they can find "local" healthy food when they're on the road. He is a super healthy guy (Nathan looks 10 years younger than he is) and he shared this thought provoking comment: "Why is it so radical to eat 'raw' vegetables when we are the only species on the entire planet that cooks our food?" We then got into a lengthy discussion about how today's food has gotten so bad compared to how it must have been 1,000 or so years ago when the soil was so much more fertile and our air and water sources virtually unpolluted. (For more information on Nathan's mission to educate people all around the world on how to eat healthy, please visit his site: http://www.nonstopawesomeness.me).

When archeologists find skulls of modern homo sapiens (thousands of years old), it's interesting that the skulls are deteriorating, but often the teeth are intact and in many cases cavity free, and in better shape than some people's teeth who are alive today! Our early ancestors didn't eat processed foods or high fructose corn syrup, snack on sugar cookies or drink sugar-laden sodas. If you've ever seen anybody with a high sugar content diet, their teeth are often full of cavities and rotting away. A dentist will tell you it is NOT the sugars that rot your teeth, but when the sugar metabolizes to acid, its the acid that creates cavities and rots your teeth. Our ancestor's diet consisted mainly of plants, nuts, berries, and a very limited amount of low fat animal protein. Cancer and other terminal illnesses were rare in part due to almost no sugar consumption.

About 2,000 years ago when grains were introduced as a cheap way to feed the masses (and vegetable & fruit intake was reduced), historians started seeing the first written records of illness and disease. The notes of early doctors documenting these sick patients are found written in stone in Egyptian Hieroglyphics. There's been a slow trend over the past few hundred years in most cultures as animals have become domesticated (especially cows, pigs, chicken, goats, sheep, etc.). Our modern day society is eating more dairy and meat products every year. There used to be conflicting messages about dairy and meat products and how they affect your health, but that is slowly changing. After reading hundreds of medical journals and books (NOT influenced by any special interest group, or industry association), it's very clear that a big part of sickness in developing countries is a direct result of the current generation eating more meat and dairy products than their grandparents. The most extensive study ever was The Atlas of Cancer Mortality in China where the Chinese Government in the 1970s employed 650,000 researchers to study 880 million people. Genetics were all the same as these were all indigenous Chinese people in similar environments and there were thousands of twins who were born and studied before the one-child policy had expanded. With meticulous research, the study came up with 94,000 direct correlations between diet and disease! This China Cancer Atlas showed cancer clusters in counties where the population had a higher intake of meat and dairy products. In one county cluster, the incidence of esophageal cancer was 400 times higher than the rest of the rural population! This is NOT a typo: that particular cancer in that specific county was 400 times higher that the other counties where virtually no meat or dairy products were consumed! [3-1]. One of the world's most recognized nutritional doctors in the world, Dr. T. Colin Campbell coordinated with the Chinese Government after this groundbreaking study, and did a follow up study in the 1980s which supported these findings. Meanwhile Dr. Caldwell Esselstyn (a world renown heart bypass surgeon) was doing his own research and shares some powerful statistics from other countries that had a plant-based diet with very little meat or dairy. In 1958 the entire country of Japan had only 18 deaths from prostrate cancer! Even though the U.S. population that year was just double that of Japan, the United States recorded 14,000 deaths from prostate cancer! In 1978 Kenya's rate of breast cancer was 82 times lower than the United States! (We all know how prevalent breast cancer is now in the U.S., just 3 decades later). In 1970, before the introduction of fast food into the

Chinese diet, the rate of heart disease was 12 times lower than in the U.S.! [3-2] You don't need to remind Dr. Esselstyn of these statistics as he was at the Cleveland Clinic performing thousands of heart bypass surgeries. Over the years, the esteemed Dr. Esselstyn finally realized that most of his patients created these heart conditions themselves and he now promotes a plant based diet and nutrition as preventative medicine. If you watch the 2011 documentary film "*Forks Over Knives*", you can see his passion for what in most cases he claims are preventable surgeries. While many of these surgeries are saving lives, they don't come cheap. The 500,000 heart bypasses every year in the U.S. now cost us over $50 billion!

One of the first radical changes to our food began in the late 1800s after Louis Pasteur invented the "pasteurization" process in France. One of the 1st products in the U.S. to be pasteurized was milk by being exposed briefly to high (often scalding) temperatures to destroy and kill microorganisms and prevent fermentation. There is often a debate about drinking pasteurized and homogenized milk as opposed to drinking raw milk coming from a small farm, grass raised dairy cow. As a utilitarian thinker most of the time, there were (and still are) benefits from pasteurization, but it is odd that humans are the only animals on the planet who: 1) drink milk from a completely different animal species and 2) keep drinking milk our entire lives after the weaning period. Now with the massive increase in dairy consumption (including milk, cream, cheese, ice cream, etc.) there have been literally thousands of studies proving that dairy foods can create all kinds of health problems from the minor food allergy to serious problems like heart disease, arthritis, and osteoporosis. This last one stuns people, but here's the TRUTH... a 12-year Harvard study of 80,000 nurses showed that a high intake of commercial milk appeared to actually increase the risk of bone fractures. Higher milk consumption (with all that great calcium medical doctors and the American Dairy Association tell us to drink every day) actually leads to higher rates of osteoporosis. [3-3] There are two reasons for this: first, when milk is pasteurized and homogenized, your body can't absorb or use all the calcium. Second, modern day milk contains animal proteins and acids which actually cause the body to leach calcium right out of the bones, but more on that in chapter 6 when we discuss acidity.

In recent history a few other major changes started happening, which increased convenience and often lowered food prices price, but diminished food quality including canned foods, which originated in France around 1800. Robert Ayars established the first American canning factory in New York City in 1812, using tin-plated wrought-iron cans for preserving meats, fruits and vegetables. Fiber and nutritional value stay pretty high in canned goods, but when extra salt or other preservatives were added, that diminished the health benefits. On a scale of 1 to 10, these canned goods delivered health benefits on the scale of an 8 or 9, but NOT quite as fresh, tasty, or healthy as eating fresh foods.

The second major change in modern day foods happened a century later with frozen food. Freezing food like fruits and vegetables was a challenge as large ice crystals would often form in the actual food damaging cell structure and not quite capturing all of the taste and freshness. In the freezing process (and later the re-heating process) more cellular damage was often done and some of the vitamins and nutrients were lost. In the 1920s Clarence Birdseye advanced the process with a high-pressure, flash-freezing technique, which did away with most of the ice crystals, and hence the major damage to the food itself. The fruits, vegetables, etc. were able to retain more of the vitamins and key nutrients. Am I saying that frozen foods are not as healthy, nutritious, and tasty as a veggie or fruit picked off the vine or tree? Yes, but that doesn't mean frozen veggies and fruits are not good for you, and I certainly would eat frozen vegetables and fruits in the "off-season" when fresh produce is not available. For many families today if frozen produce is cheaper (which it often is), this a great second option, but when fresh food is available and affordable, it's common sense that exposing the produce to extreme temperatures on both ends and physically changing the food's "state" is NOT 100% as good as eating fresh.

One of the few orthodox medical doctors in the 1950s and 1960s who became very outspoken (and often criticized by his peers for his view on how important food was as medicine) was Dr. Henry Bieler who in 1966 published Food is Your Best Medicine. Since this book is based on lasting results, I mention the fact that he noticed his energy levels seemed to be decreasing during his long work hours at his practice, and he over the years had gained a significant amount of weight. He went on a mostly alkaline diet cutting out sugars & starches, salt, all drugs, and limiting animal proteins. In less than a year, Dr. Beiler went from 210 to 137 lbs. and dramatically raised his energy and vitality. Most importantly, he kept that weight off for years practicing what he preached. Dr. Beiler later became a Chair of Nutrition at Columbia University and a Chair of Dietetic Medicine at Columbia University's Goldwater Memorial Hospital.

Other radical trends in food (especially here in the U.S.) started changing in the 1950s after World War II. As our country developed, so did the advent of massive grocery stores where millions could walk down the aisles and for the first time pick up frozen "TV dinners", canned meats, processed cereals, or other packaged foods with additives and preservatives. In the 1960s and 1970s the fast food restaurant craze spread like wildfire with major chains like McDonald's and Burger King changing the way Americans ate all around the country. In addition to the fast food phenomenon, the U.S. started massive corn subsidies and with along with cheap refined corn chips and other products, high fructose corn syrup was developed which became an inexpensive substitute for sugar and was added to hundreds of different food products.

The advent of microwave ovens in the 1970s provided convenience to hard working families everywhere and reinforced the convenience of processed, packaged, or frozen meals that could be cooked or reheated in seconds, once again pushing whole foods like farm fresh vegetables to the back of the grocery cart.

Factory farming continued to expand in the 1970s and 1980s and eventually when the animals started to get sicker and sicker from cramped quarters, antibiotics were introduced as well as cheap corn feed, and later steroids and growth hormones. Higher doses of antibiotics, steroids, and super growth hormones have helped raise cattle, pigs, and chickens in record time and have miraculously kept the cost of a hamburger down to 99 cents or less the past decade!

On top of all this, the past 15 years have seen deep school budget cuts which have spurred school districts to take money from soda companies on campus (soda vending machines can generate lots of extra revenues), as can allowing vendors like Taco Bell & Pizza Hut to service the lunch menu for kids. All of these factors have made our food less "natural" and more acidic (as described in chapter 6). If you've been to an elementary school recently and seen the growing number of obese, sick looking kids you now know why. Energy drinks are also a disturbing trend with new brands flooding the market every year. Consider the alarming fact that one 24 oz. Monster Energy Drink ® contains 240mg of caffeine. That is seven (7) times the amount of caffeine in one 12 oz. can of Coke! While there is evidence that these energy drinks may have caused over a dozen deaths and over 7,000 emergency room visits, kids are still drinking these elixirs like crazy. To any logical parent reading this, I would NOT let my kid drink any energy drinks!

The latest controversy is over genetically modified (or "biotech") foods. These foods are derived from genetically modified organisms (GMOs), such as genetically modified crops including corn, soybeans, and cotton now prevalent in the U.S. GMOs have specific changes introduced into their DNA by genetic engineering techniques. While there are some advantages to GMO foods such as lower food costs, and in some cases larger crop yields, there is plenty of controversy and lots of unanswered questions about these new foods, which were introduced in the 1990s. Many countries in Europe & Asia have banned GM foods and other countries that have allowed limited GM foods usually require a labeling system that informs consumers whether or not they're eating all natural food or genetically modified ("altered") food. An example is rGBH (a growth hormone injected in cows) in widespread use in the U.S., but banned in 27 other countries after studies linked rGBH to breast cancer increases (7 times more likely) and prostate cancer (4 times more likely). [3-4] William Lee Cowden, M.D. (a cardiologist and internist) teaches other doctors and patients to "avoid all GMO foods." [3-5]. Until the verdict is out, I do my best to avoid foods that I know are modified and where possible buy products like Silk™ brand soymilk (which is voluntarily labeled as GMO-free). On another note about GMOs, when I was a kid, it was extremely rare that anybody in school had any food allergies. I remember only (1) classmate out of 40 + kids in our 2nd grade class who had an allergy to milk and the teacher made a really big deal about it. These days, it's not uncommon for 25% of the kids in elementary school to come in with a laundry list of different foods they are allergic to! This trend has really disturbed me and I recently came across this statistic provided by a RN who runs a modern health blog. "In the last twenty years, there has been an epidemic increase in allergies, asthma, and auto-immune disorders. Today, it is estimated that 20% of American children have allergies, and that there has been a 400% increase in food allergies, a 300% increase in asthma, with a 56% increase in asthma deaths"! [3-6] I would strongly recommend that you watch the new documentary film "Genetic Roulette: The Gamble of Our Lives" if you want to learn more. To me, there are far too many unanswered questions to be eating GMO food especially since so many other countries (with healthier populations than the U.S.) have banned GMOs.

Our food did not get this bad overnight, but over the past 30 – 40 years especially, our food that the general population consumes today is really, really BAD! It makes more sense than ever to educate yourself and eat the best food you can.

BONUS CHAPTER: Pour Some SUGAR On Me!

Just like the 1987 hit song "Pour Some Sugar on Me!" by Def Leppard, it seems today, we're drowning in sugar. This was an additional chapter relevant in the Alkalize section, because excess sugar metabolizes to acid and is now one of the biggest problems in the U.S. today. BusinessInsider.com found that in 2010 the average American ate over 100 lbs. of sugar every year! [3-7] WholeVegan.com did a more recent study that showed that over 50% of Americans now eat 180 lbs. of sugar each year! That is quite an increase from the18 lbs. of processed sugar people in this country ate just 200 years ago. This sugar craze usually starts with getting children hooked on sugar (which dietary experts have called an "addictive drug"). Children watching cartoons see dozens of cereal commercials every Saturday morning and when they travel in tow with their parents to the grocery store, many of the kid's cereals are located on the lower shelves easy for children to spot. Most parents would never dream of feeding Twinkies or several slices of chocolate fudge cake to their children first thing in the morning before school, but with some cereals having 20 grams of sugar per cup, this is what they are doing. I've witnessed children having at least two (2) medium sized bowls of cereal (remember sugar is addictive & tastes so good) which would start your child off with 60 grams of sugar from the cereal alone. The flavored (or even worse chocolate) milk can add another 28 grams of sugar. If your child has juice, today's "juice" drink (only 15% juice, but labeled similar to real juice and cheaper), can add another 30 grams of sugar. Many of the children's vitamins now have glucose syrup or sorbitol (an added sugar substitute), so that's even more sugar! If your child just has just 2 bowls of cereal, some juice and a vitamin, he or she could easily start off the morning with almost 130 grams of sugar, let alone 500+ empty calories to help jump start child obesity. This is absolute insanity! Sugar (or sugar substitutes) are in almost every single food item you see in the grocery store. Just look at the following table to see how the sugar all adds up:

BREAKFAST ITEM	AMOUNT of SUGAR
1 bowl of Kellogg's Sugar Smacks Cereal	20 grams
½ cup flavored milk	28 grams
2nd bowl of cereal	20 grams
½ cup flavored milk	28 grams
Juice "Drink"	30 grams
Multi-Vitamin	3 grams
TOTAL	**129 grams!**

This should be a wake up call for you and your children (if you have any). Of course this assumes your child does not add a couple of slices of toast (loaded with artificial butter & sugar laden jelly). This also assumes your kid would not be one of the millions of kids who grabs a soda and candy bar from the school vending machines later that morning when the 1st sugar crash hits a few hours after his or her nutritional breakfast. No wonder the Centers for Disease Control in 2011 classified 17% of American children classified as obese, and some other studies have estimated 33% of teenagers and adolescents are now obese. Many experts are seriously concerned that this obesity number could approach 50% of all American children in the next 5 – 10 years! A recent Pediatrics report found that overall, half of overweight teens and have one or more risk factors for heart disease, diabetes, high blood pressure, or high levels of bad cholesterol. [3-8]

They say a picture is worth a thousand words, so here's a visual analogy how sugar burns in the human body... Think about an open campfire that already has a flame going. If you were to pour gasoline directly onto that fire, those flames would immediately flare up, providing you with beautiful colors with lots of light and warmth for a few seconds, and then the flames will quickly die down. That gasoline is similar to you slugging a sugar-laden soda. You will immediately get a great sugar high; feel great for a few seconds, but it won't last long. Now visualize the fire again... if you've placed some small kindling (my favorite is tiny dead pine branches with lots of bark & sap) on a fire, this too will flame up almost like gasoline giving you a bright large flame, lots of heat for a few minutes longer this time, but eventually the fire will soon die down. The only way to build a long lasting, steady fire is once the fire is going add some large logs (dry, "dead" oak is particularly good) that will burn steady, slow and last a long time. The next time you are by a campfire, or even a regular fireplace notice the size of the large logs that are burning for a long time. Now lets look at the calories (fyi…calories like the fire represent "heat energy" that your body burns) you are putting into your body every day. If you are eating foods with mostly sugar (or even $1/3^{rd}$ of your calorie intake is sugar), you are definitely experiencing sugar highs & lows let alone all the long-term health risks. Why not visualize the steady, long burning fireplace and give your body the long lasting fuel (protein & carbohydrates, with a small mix of natural fat & sugar) to perform consistently. A few examples of breakfast foods that have much lower sugar content (while also being healthier) would include: organic soy or almond milk, 100% fruit or vegetable juice, organic eggs, nuts, wheat toast (without jelly), yogurt, vegetables, or fruit (a limited amount as most fruit is high in sugar). At the end of the book, you'll find a few recipes for some easy to make, healthy, nutritious breakfast smoothies.

"When it comes to eating right & exercising, there is no 'I'll start tomorrow.' Tomorrow is disease!"
- V.L. Allineare

CHAPTER FOUR (4):
Dr. Young's Fishbowl Analogy

Back in the 1800s, doctors and biologists always thought that disease and sickness came from germs and viruses outside the body that attack and make individuals sick. Even today, there are many traditionally trained M.D.'s who still talk to their patients in this manner and have the philosophy that in order for their patients to stay healthy, they must ward off these outside germs by taking flu shots, take preventative medications and at the 1st hint of sickness, of course take more prescriptions including antibiotics. To the contrary, most nutritionists (and medical doctors with an extensive preventative medicine background) argue that the BEST way to fend off sickness is to have a super healthy and strong immune system.

One of the modern day pioneers who has focused on alkalizing the body as the best way to perfect health is Dr. Robert O. Young. Dr. Young is now recognized as one of the top research scientists in the world and throughout his career, his research has been focused at the cellular level. His premise is that if your body is properly alkalized and at the optimal pH level (around 7.36), just as your optimal body temperature should be close to 98.6, the human body will function perfectly and be able to cure itself and maintain homeostasis. Neil Solomon, M.D., Ph.D. Former Head of Research for John Hopkins University has the highest praise for Dr. Young stating: "Dr. Young may be on the threshold of a new biology, whose principle—if proven—could revolutionize the biology and medicine worlds".

One of the best visuals to keeping your body healthy is Dr. Young's "Fishbowl Water" analogy. Most of us have had goldfish (or some other pet fish) at one point in time. Dr. Young's analogy is very simple, but profound. He explains: "Think of the importance of maintaining the integrity of the internal fluids of the body that we 'swim' in daily. Imagine the fish in this tank are your cells and organ systems bathed in fluids, which transport food and remove wastes. Now imagine we back up a car and put the tailpipe up against the air intake filter that supplies the oxygen for the water in the tank instead of a quality water machine. The water becomes filled with carbon monoxide, lowering the alkaline pH, creating an acidic pH environment, and threatening the health of the 'fish', your cells and organs." [4-1] Even a child who has ever had a goldfish, is very careful to not overfeed his or her pet (which would create excess acids, etc.), and if the bowl or tank does not have a filtration system, that same kid would learn to always change the water out every so often so that the fish is not "polluted" by its own excrement, algae growth, etc. Unfortunately some people who have fish, see their pet(s) die if they don't feed the fish enough (starvation), or more commonly if the water becomes too toxic. Any person who has fish and notices that their fish is not swimming well, or looks sluggish or sickly, the first thing they do is change the water! Isn't it common sense that we should also regularly cleanse our bodies (including our intestines and colons) and make sure the food and drinks we put into our bodies is healthy (and for the most part alkaline)? As tragic as it is in today's society (and the main reason the U.S. has the "sickest" population in the world), we tend to rush to the doctor to get a pill or ask about a treatment or surgery. As a business, traditional doctors, hospitals, and pharmaceutical companies would go broke if those institutions sent all of their customers home and told them to try the homeopathic method of curing themselves by alkalizing. Medical doctors get paid for seeing more patients, writing prescription drugs, and performing procedures. Hospitals make money running expensive tests and scans (very often unnecessary) and performing surgeries. Now I am NOT suggesting that you stop visiting your doctor, or stop taking prescription drugs cold turkey, or put off necessary tests and ignore life saving surgeries, but doesn't it make sense to look at the water in the fishbowl first? Look at the food you are eating and your body's environment very carefully as that is your "fishbowl". I encourage you to visit Dr. Young's website (www.pHMiracleLiving.com) to read more on this as well as his extensive research on the subject of alkalinity. On Dr. Young's website, there is an excellent short video describing this critical concept. Here's another common sense analogy to ponder. No reasonable person who owns an automobile would stop doing oil changes every 5,00 miles (along with a semi-regular engine flush, and oil filter change) to keep the car running efficiently. The healthiest people I know and have studied (who never get sick) usually do some sort of cleanse or detox once a year. I will cover the 7-Day "Alkalize & Energize" cleanse in great details later on as well as in the Appendix of this book. For now though, keep reading and in the next chapter you will learn a lot more about alkalinity and why this is the most important concept to your health and the longevity of your life!

"Sometimes I wake up in the morning & go Ahh...I don't want to work out! But I do anyway, because I'll always feel better afterwards. I have NEVER once worked out & felt worse!"
- Actress & Activist Alexandra Paul

CHAPTER FIVE (5): Introduction to Alkalinity

While I've been doing several years of research and am in development on a feature length companion documentary "Do These Things or You Will Die" film (which should be released next year), the best introduction I got to the importance of Alkalinity was from my friend Tony Robbins. Tony who has a CD program called "Get the Edge" and one of the sessions is all about Alkalinity and how it changed his life and his understanding of health, disease, cancer, etc. I strongly recommend this program "Get the Edge" or you may be able to find it at your local library. It is the most logical, simple, and profound introduction to this critically important topic of Alkalinity. Tony is a master at synthesizing information (in this case from doctors, nutritionists, and other health experts) and explaining any subject in layman's terms. My company, Nemours Marketing did our own follow up research (from over books & dozens of interviews, etc.) before alkalizing different people with our 7-Day "Alkalize & Energize" cleanse (over 50 people to date), some of whose amazing results are shared in this book. As mentioned previously, 7.36 is the ideal pH level your body should be (which is slightly alkaline), or your body will literally break itself down, leading to illness, disease, and cancer. Healthy, "alkaline" cells have lots of electrons (which provide electrical energy) and ensure a negative charge on your red blood cells which help them move swiftly & efficiently through the blood stream. Dr. Robert Young wrote a comprehensive book on this subject called The pH Miracle. What Dr. Young shares from all his research is that obese people are usually "over-acid". On CNN, he showed remarkable photos of some of his patients who have lost over 100 lbs. and are now totally healthy. More and more doctors like Dr. Leonard Coldwell (www.DrLeonardColdwell.com) are stating that cancer can be stopped completely by fully alkalizing your body. Tony Robbins himself is the poster boy for perfect health as he spends as many as 275 days on the road each year meeting tens of thousands of people. You could not be more exposed to more germs or potentially sick people than Tony, yet he consistently has such incredible energy & has never been sick in over 25 years! Tony will attribute his incredible energy, vitality, and health to his alkaline diet and lifestyle.

My simple analogy of the importance of 7.36 pH alkalinity is the 98.6 degrees Fahrenheit that your body should function at. If you are outside on a super hot day, certain body functions will slow down, blood flow to your extremities will increase, and your body will start sweating. On a very cold day, your body will limit the amount of blood flowing to your outer epidermis (your skin) and eventually your muscles will contract as you start shivering. This involuntary action of shivering is to keep your body moving and therefore warm your body is also a warning signal to do something like light a fire, find shelter, or add clothing to warm your body up. Your body is smart enough to also warn you of increased acidity. If your body falls much below the 7.36 pH balance level, you can get ulcers, acid reflux, stomach aches, feel fatigued, just to name a few warning signals. It is absolutely ridiculous to keep ignoring these signals to the body! The solution is not just to take more Tums, Alka-Seltzer, or Prilosec. This would be like driving your car and the yellow engine light comes on and instead of changing the motor oil, the oil filter, the air filter and giving the car a tune up, you instead cut the little wire to the dashboard light and keep on driving... sooner or later you're going to pay the piper. This is exactly what happens when we too often ignore all the signals of an acidic body. In just a few months, or a few years disease will appear or worse some kind of cancer when often it is too late. Just like battery acid that spills onto your battery post and starts corroding the battery terminals, too much acid in your body will start corroding your organs and disrupting all kinds of body functions leading to a complete breakdown of normal body functions as you'll learn in the next chapter.

In 1994, Dr. Young discovered the biological transformation of red blood cells into bacteria in acidic environments. Dr. Young and his wife Shelley as mentioned are alkalinity experts and have written many other books on the subject of alkalinity and Ph balance. Their noble life mission is to do all they can to change lives and save lives with an alkaline lifestyle and diet. Finally almost 3 decades later for his ground breaking work on alkalinity, Dr. Young is starting to get the respect he deserves from some of his peers such as this quote from Neil Solomon, M.D., Ph.D: "Dr.Young may be on the threshold of a new biology whose principles will revolutionize the biology and medicine worlds."

The patient should be made to understand that he or she must take charge of his own life. Don't take your body to the doctor as if he were a repair shop.
- Quentin Regestein

CHAPTER SIX (6): All About ACID...
the Cause of Cancer, Sickness, and Disease!

The **most important section of this book** (and what has changed my health the most) **is the concept of "Alkalizing" your body**. Understanding the delicate pH balance of your body and the effect acid has is critical. If you read the book Alkalize or Die by Dr. Theodore A. Baroody, you'll understand that managing the pH balance in your body and limiting your acid is a matter of life and death! If you think I'm being dramatic here, look around at your family & friends and see if any of them have any life threatening diseases, major illnesses, or cancer. Ask yourself if more people you know are battling arthritis, osteoporosis, or general body pains the past few years? The health epidemic for these ailments in the U.S. is growing out of control as is obesity. I recently heard that the U.S. was the "fattest" country in the world and figured the average American citizen was maybe 4 or 5 lbs. heavier than the average citizen from other countries. I was stunned to read the latest weight study revealed by Time Magazine stated the "average U.S. person weighs in at 180 lbs. (outweighing the rest of the world by 43 lbs. per person)"! [6-1] As mentioned, my friend Tony Robbins explains in plain English how acid destroys your body starting at the cellular level with your blood cells. Tony has spent several decades studying, researching, and speaking to the world's top experts in blood, cellular health, energy, and nutrition. Tony's explanation will paint a visual picture for you and help you truly understand alkalinity and encourage you to take action towards perfect health. When several family members and friends died of cancer the last few years, that was a real wake up call for me. After my college roommate and fraternity brother (John Clark) died way too young from cancer, I watched a life changing film called "The Gerson Miracle" which is now available on NetFlix or for free on many internet channels. Dr. Max Gerson was a ground breaking German physician who developed The Gerson Therapy (an all natural alternative dietary therapy), and in 1958 published a book in which he documented curing 50 terminal cancer patients: A Cancer Therapy: Results of 50 Cases. The ground-breaking work that Dr. Gerson started is now continued by his daughter Charlotte Gerson and delivers proven results! The success rate the Gerson clinics has is astounding, and you can read direct testimonials from dozens of cancer survivors including people like Susan Morton who share their stories at www.Gerson.org. This legendary clinic now has recovered cancer patients surviving decades after they were sentenced by Medical Doctors to just a few months left to live! Unfortunately the American Medical Association and the FDA will not let these treatments continue in the United States, so Charlotte Gerson opened a clinic in Mexico (just south of their San Diego headquarters) and a clinic in Hungary. The whole premise of Dr. Gerson's work and the book Alkalize or Die is that once a body becomes acidic, it will start breaking down almost everything starting at the cellular level. Problems may start slowly like fatigue (most American's can relate to this), allergies, acid reflux, sicknesses (including colds and flu symptoms), disease, and eventually cancer. Another main side effect of a body being too acidic is obesity. As explained in an earlier chapter, the pH scale goes from 0 – 14 with 7 being neutral and your body's pH should be slightly alkaline at 7.36. Once your body gets lower than 7.36 (slightly acidic), all sorts of problems start occurring including obesity. Here's the simple explanation why acidity directly leads to obesity. Your body runs on electricity (starting with your heart which is an electrical pump) and every part of your body is connected by your nervous system's electric grid. Individual nerve cells (called neurons) send signals to other cells as electrochemical waves traveling along thin fibers called axons, so if you stub your toe within a fraction of a second, this information is relayed to your brain which causes you to feel pain and shout "ouch". Now back to the acid problem in our diets and how it leads to obesity. Your body is extremely sophisticated and has a defense mechanism built in to protect your bones and all of your vital organs. When any excess acid is detected (once your ph level gets below 7.36), your body's neurons alert the brain "Hey body... we have too much acid and it looks like there is more acid entering the body... holy crap... danger! We just got an alert that another 64 oz. soda is streaming down the esophagus." What happens next is a survival mechanism: your body starts retaining more & more fat to protect your skeletal system, your vital organs, and inner workings of your body from all that acid. As Dr. Robert Young explains in his book The pH Miracle, obesity is not just created by people eating too much (although taking in more calories than you burn each day will also lead to becoming overweight), but by people being "too acidic".[6-2] About 15 years ago when I first started researching the ph balance and this acidity problem, I had an incredible epiphany that I remember to this day. I used to go Bally's gym on a regular basis (at least once a week) and there were a few people at the gym who worked out almost every day. I noticed one gentleman named Justin in particular who was hard core on the treadmill (he huffed & puffed for a good hour) and then on certain days Justin would work different parts of his body including upper body, lower body, medicine balls and even advanced aerobics class for an extreme cardio workout. Other days he would run 5 miles on the indoor track sprinting the last ¼ mile. Justin bragged about having a good diet and that he did not drink alcohol or smoke, and he was in his early 30s. Justin was in good overall shape, but for the amount of effort he invested, he should have had a "six pack" stomach and V-shaped torso that you see on professional swimmers or Olympic athletes. Instead Justin had two small "love handles" on either side of his hips. I bet that 95% of all the guys over the age of 35 reading this book can relate to those damn love handles that never seem to go away no matter how much and how hard they work out. For ladies over 40, there is the dreaded rear end (butt pad) or the very top back portion of your legs that seems to collect cellulite. Even for people in good shape, it can be maddening to have those extra 2- 3 lbs. or for some people maybe the extra 5 – 10 lbs. of excess fat in those places that never, ever seems to go away! Well the "ah-ha" moment for me happened one day after I watched Justin finish a 60 minute treadmill session followed by 30 minutes of core body work out including crunches, sit ups, leg lifts, etc. Justin waved good-bye and seemed proud about completing another intense work out. When he walked through the lobby, he stopped at the vending machine and bought a large bottle of Mountain Dew! Eureka... the light bulb went off in my head that even though Justin said he had a healthy diet, worked out like a maniac 5 – 6 days a week, he was dumping liquid acid (and excess sugar) into his body after his workouts. No wonder Justin could never get rid of his love handles! After more reading, research, and dozens of trials of clients I've consulted with, the answer to million dollar question everybody is dying to know: "**How can I possibly get rid of my last few lbs. of unwanted fat?**" The undisputed **answer** in all of our research and that we have proven with over 50 clients so far is to **eliminate the ACID!** A few of my initial clients included actors who needed to lose 10 – 15 lbs. in a 1 week time frame for film roles. I am not bragging to try and impress you, but honestly want to impress upon you that MOST people can lose a significant amount of weight (including toxins stored in their bodies) in a very short period of time simply by alkalizing their bodies.

Speaking of working out, there is a major trap that many fitness buffs fall into these days which is the new Protein bars. Protein bars are a booming business with dozens of brands out now and here's the HUGE PROBLEM with most of them. They are loaded with way TOO MUCH protein! If you snack on a protein bar that has 28 – 35 grams of protein, and you eat that bar in one sitting as most people do, that is over twice as much protein as your body can assimilate. The excess protein actually becomes an acid ash. I've even seen well meaning parents send their kids off to school with these mega protein bars and once again, there is no possible way a small kid's body can assimilate that much protein at one time. So this whole "Protein Hype" is great marketing and a scam to sell more protein bars. Once you complete the 7-Day "Alkalize & Energize" cleanse, the best and most healthy diet lifestyle long term is a balance of protein, carbohydrates with a small amount of fats. Yes... fat! Another false hype is all these foods that are "fat free!". This is another scam to sell more processed food, but in reality a little bit of fat in your diet is not only good for you, but essential to your good health. You have probably heard about really healthy people including most athletes eating a well balanced diet and also eating 4 (or sometimes 5) smaller meals throughout the day. Just like overloading your body with a mega-protein bar at one sitting is bad for you, eating smaller well-balanced meals is also easier on your digestive system. This should make more sense to you than eating a huge dinner and lunch or having a late night pig out session in front of the television. I'll cover more on this balance later on in the book.

Meanwhile, contributing author Ronald Farnham has been experimenting with us for two (2) years now and while he lost 60 lbs. in 90 days simply by alkalizing (90% of his diet was vegetable juice). Ronald's "before & after" photos are pretty amazing and his story will also be in the upcoming documentary film we'll be releasing in the near future. As Ronald mentioned in his chapter, without excessive exercise (no running, weight lifting, P-90X, etc.) but just by alkalizing his system the weight fell off his body like butter. There were several days on his weight loss tracking sheet (very important to have this as well as a target weight "goal"), Ronald lost 2 or 3 lbs! I once lost 20 lbs. in 7 days on one of my cleanses. What's really interesting is that every single time (without exception) that Ronald had a strenuous workout like pitching an entire baseball game (Ronald used to be a professional baseball player), his weight loss would stop for 1 or 2 days due to build up of lactic acid! At the end of my 7 day "alkaline & energize" cleanse, I decided to keep juicing for 1 more day, but also decided to lift some weights and also run 4 miles including some wind sprints to the point of muscle fatigue. The next day instead of the scale reading 1 – 2 lbs. less, I was shocked as I had gained 1.5 lbs! Here is the critical point to learn here. **Doing strenuous exercise or massive workouts will NOT help you lose weight as you are creating additional lactic acid.** In fact, we tell people during the 7-day "Alkalize & Energize" cleanse NOT to do any major exercise! I don't mean to keep beating a dead horse here, but millions of Americans are facing major obesity with the many more having the allergies, sickness, disease, and cancer that often goes along with being overweight. Another problem of an acidic body is the candida (yeast) which as many as 90% of Americans have in their systems. Candida feed on glucose, so this is where the constant "sugar cravings" come from. The constant cravings for sugar, sweets, coffee, and in some cases alcohol can be eliminated once you kill off the candidia by alkalizing your system! Don't you want to stop this vicious cycle of overeating, being overweight, and not having lots of energy? On the weight issue, be honest with yourself! Whether you are 10 lbs. overweight or 50 lbs. overweight, doing our 7-Day "Alkalize & Energize" cleanse outlined in this book will start you losing weight immediately and give you more energy. If you don't lose weight and you don't feel an improved energy level simply write us and ask for 100% of your money back! It doesn't matter if you bought this book on Amazon, in a bookstore, or on the NemoursMarketing.com website. Just send us your purchase receipt and return book and we'll issue you a 100% refund, no questions asked!

With the massive increase in processed foods with added sugars, salts, artificial flavors, colorings, & preservatives, it's not hard to figure out why most people in the U.S. are not nearly as healthy as the previous generation. We already discussed the dramatically increased cancer rate (in just the past 30 years), but going back to weight, I was at the famous Griffith Park carousel (you've seen in dozens of movies) last week where the park preserved the old carousel just like it was back in the 1960s & 70s. I noticed a sign that read: "weight limit for riders is 200 lbs." If Disney World posted a sign like that on any of their rides I would imagine 25% of all the Dads would not be able to go on the rides with their kids. I know for a fact there are a few ladies out there and some teenage kids who also exceed the 200lb. weight limit, so they too would not be allowed to have fun on the rides if we upheld the same standards we had a few years ago.

Getting back to acid (since it is the root cause of obesity, many diseases, & cancer), I want to briefly discuss meat (which contains uric acid) as one of my friend's beliefs about meat are not entirely accurate. One of my friend's claims: "We were born carnivores and we need red meat for protein to stay healthy." Science and history prove something quite different. If you look at early cavemen (homo erectus and the earliest forms of homo sapiens), our mutual ancestors were designed to eat mostly organic plants, vegetables, berries, and sprouts. We were never designed to eat meat (as mentioned, loaded with uric acid), especially the huge quantity of meat most Americans eat now at every single meal. Don't believe me? Why then do we not have fangs or any teeth (like big cats, bears, wolves, etc.) to tear and shred meat with? Why don't we have any claws or appendices to fight & kill other animals? Why don't we have 4 legs to propel us quick enough to catch other fast animals? Why don't we have super keen sense of smell that most other predators have? And most importantly, why do humans have an incredibly long and twisted intestine & colon (obviously never meant to digest large quantities of meat)? Long before man evolved with his large brain and started developing spears, knives and other hunting tools man lived off of plants including vegetables, fruits, berries, and nuts. Coming back to present day, everyone knows that eating green leafy vegetables are healthy & the best source of nutrition, vitamins, calcium, minerals, and overall health, but it is astonishing how little greens are in most people's diets. Despite what most American school children think, ketchup is not a vegetable and neither are French fries or potato chips. The frozen vegetables people grab at the grocery or convenience stores and then microwave for dinner are not much better since they've been depleted of some of their vitamins, minerals and other nutritional content. A certain amount of raw, uncooked, unprocessed vegetables is key to long lasting health. This would include fresh salads, juiced vegetables (not store bought in a can), and the "green" powdered drink, which will be discussed in chapter 9.

I could list dozens of stories where acidic diets create havoc with people's bodies and their well-being many of which were among the 12,000 people I spoke to at the Medco table. Here is one other shocking story, which I came across today while working on a TV show. I met with an absolutely gorgeous girl named Stacey who is strikingly beautiful and a very lean body. Stacey mentioned that she was 5' 7" and weighed about 115 lbs. There was no indication at all that she had any health issues. It turns out that this 37 years "young" girl has some allergies, but also some serious arthritis! In cold weather especially, it is troublesome as she does not have great circulation in her hands and feet and her doctor confirmed that she did in fact have arthritis. I asked if she had ever seen photos of her blood (not just a typical blood report from the lab). With new optical high definition microscopes you can now see how healthy your blood is and get an idea if it is "acidic", or healthy and "alkaline". I had a hunch that she might have been eating a few acidic items on a regular basis. Turns out, she is a "meat & potatoes" gal and eats chicken or red meat on a fairly regular basis, potatoes, pasta, and the occasional soda. While she does eat a limited amount of salads or vegetables, she admitted later that alkaline veggies do not make up even 50% of her diet. Having even a slightly acidic system is a recipe for disaster. Hopefully by the time you read this book, Stacey will have done the 7-Day "Alkalize & Energize" cleanse and decides to reclaim her health. I truly want to help people like Stacey and if we can get rid of any signs of arthritis that she has now, we'll be sure to include that health miracle in the documentary film companion to this book.

I had an extended interview with Dr. M. Phyllis Lose (the legendary equine veterinarian whose life is chronicled in the best selling book No Job For a Lady). Although Dr. Lose is in her mid-80s and technically retired, she is a "model" for perfect health as she already does most of the tips in this book and she still works vaccinating animals waking up Saturdays and Sundays at 4:30am to work for her clients and making life pleasant for the thousands of animals (mostly horses) she has treated over her 60 year career. When we started discussing diet and alkalinity, she brought up an interesting point that there was NO insurance for animals years ago like there is medical insurance for us. Although there is now pet insurance (even for dogs and cats since they are now ironically getting affected by more cancer and terminal diseases), the owners of the horses Dr. Lose would examine including thoroughbreds for racing or breeding demanded the best food to ensure that their investment (very expensive horses) stayed healthy. Dr. Lose did perform quite a few surgeries and in fact as the 1st female equine veterinarian in the U.S., she pioneered some of the modern day surgical techniques. Dr. Lose found the most effective way to keep a horse healthy was to get the perfect blend of alfalfa, green timothy, and clover. The perfect blend of these highly alkaline foods could slow down and in many cases prevent arthritis and osteoporosis. Another interesting note is whenever the top racehorses got stomach ulcers (either from the stress of racing or the lactic acid that is physically produced inside the horse's body when racing), she had a fail proof solution... just treat the horse with sodium bicarbonate (which is an alkaline drink - technically an antacid). Voila, after a few swigs of that sodium bicarbonate, the horse's ulcer goes away and often times joint pain also subsides very quickly.

Referring specifically to the milk discussion in chapter 3, higher milk consumption (with all that great calcium medical doctors and the American Dairy Association tell us to drink every day) actually leads to higher rates of osteoporosis! Part of this is due to the animal proteins and acids which actually cause the body to leach calcium right out of the bones and the second problem is that even pure raw, organic milk from another animal species that has never been homogenized or pasteurized is NOT the best source of calcium. Just think about where the cow got the calcium in the first place? It was from the green grasses including the alkaline timothy, clover, and alfalfa. Humans can get great calcium right from the source from greens especially spinach, kale, wheat grass, etc. which are all alkaline. I can't begin to tell you how many people I've talked to who walked up to the Medco table complaining of bone loss and osteoporosis. While most are older people in their 60s, 70s, and 80s, they have this blind faith that if they keep drinking 3 glasses of milk a day and take extra calcium pills their bone density loss will decrease. The ONLY people I've ever met with (either at the Medco table or off duty) who do not have an osteoporosis problem are vegetarians. Commons sense would say they are getting plenty of calcium right from the plant source and since they don't have the extra dairy acids, the body has plenty of alkalinity, it is does NOT have to leach the bones of its calcium and other minerals. I want to make an important point here and I am NOT saying to stop drinking milk. However if you have been losing bone density over the past year and have not been able to reverse or at least stop the loss, please research this acidity concept. Doing the same thing over and over and expecting different results is INSANITY! The same goes for arthritis. It has been stated in many research articles that drinking milk can cause inflammation of the joints and lead to arthritis. Of course any other acidic foods like coffee sodas, refined foods with sugars can also lead to arthritis. Having any kind of joint pain, swelling, stiffness, and limited movement is a horrible way to live the final 20 – 30 years of your life. The good news is that more and more doctors and nutrition experts are proving that even rheumatoid arthritis (in which the body's own immune system starts to attack body tissues around joints) can be minimized and in many cases reversed with an alkaline diet and muscular therapy. Dr. Lose mentioned an interesting comment in passing that she has observed her entire career in treating thousands of animals. She stated (and this applies to people as well): "What keeps us alive is our strong immune system." Almost ALL doctors will agree that the quickest way to wreck havoc on your immune system by letting it become acid. After you finish reading this section you need to determine are you going to be among the 99% who take the Tums, the Alka-Seltzer, the Zantac or the Prilosec pill, which are all treating the symptoms of acidity? Or are you going to be among the 1% who want to get to the root cause of these problems and alkalize, so that your immune system and all of your internal organs start working again in harmony?

One medical professional (Patty Kay) who has seen just about every single illness and disease you could find in a hospital, actually worked in a hospital as a registered nurse (R.N.) for almost 40 years. I met Patty and her daughter Vanessa on a commercial shoot where we spent the majority of the day (almost 12 hours) discussing alkalinity. Patty and her daughter are both in amazing health as they are vegetarians and try to always eat organic. Patty had recently quit the nursing industry out of frustration and disgust with the protocol the hospitals and doctors would issue to recovering cancer patients. Patty was flabbergasted that in this day and age that patients with cancer were given eggs, bacon, orange juice, coffee, toast, and jelly. While these items are part of the SAD (Sad American Diet), these are all acidic foods, which would only add to the toxins already in the patient's bodies who were doing chemotherapy or radiation treatments. If Patty were able to talk to any of the patients, she would have recommended alkaline foods, vegetable juices, lemon water, and green tea. After seeing hundreds of patients die in the hospital while at the same time dozens of her friends outside the hospital doing holistic cancer treatments lived and thrived, she finally quit.

Coming up in chapter 11, you'll find a detailed list of illnesses, diseases, and medical conditions that in most cases can be reversed or minimized with an alkaline diet. If you contact the Gerson Institute directly, you'll see undisputed evidence of the worst cancer cases that have been treated successfully! I initially thought the title of Baroody's book Alkalize or Die was a little dramatic, but it isn't at all. Keep reading and you'll understand that if you don't do all the key things in this book (most importantly getting rid of the excess acids & toxins in your system) you will have a much better chance of dying sooner rather than later!

"He who takes medicine and neglects to diet
wastes the skill of his doctors."
- Chinese Proverb

CHAPTER SEVEN (7): Toxins and Poisons

The Merriam-Webster definition of toxic is: "containing or being poisonous material especially when capable of causing death or serious debilitation (eg. *toxic* waste)." A toxin then is defined as: "a poisonous substance that is a specific product of the metabolic activities of a living organism and is usually very unstable, notably toxic when introduced into the tissues, and typically capable of inducing antibody formation." [7-1] Compared to just 100 years ago, when there were a handful of chemicals, there are now close to 100,000 man made chemicals with 1,000 or more new ones introduced each year, many of which are harmful to have contact with your skin, breathe, or eat. These toxic materials, poisons, or chemicals can weaken your immune system making it even more important today to eat as many natural, organic, healthy foods as possible.

If you examine the composition of the human body (specifically a child's body) that has not had any toxins or poisons introduced to it, it's composed of 75 – 80% water while the brain is as much as 85% water. Therefore **it's common sense that MOST of what we should consume is pure, clean water and water-soluble foods such as vegetables, fruits, and sprouts!** Instead, most people in the U.S. consume soda, flavored juice & tea drinks, coffee, energy drinks, and the new craze "flavored" water beverages. These drinks are not a substitute for pure water (what your body is composed of and really needs) and in fact as you learned in earlier chapters these beverages (just like alcohol) are acidic. As you learned in chapter 3, the preponderance of sugar most Americans consume is like dumping straight acid & toxins into our body along with other artificial colorings & flavorings, processed foods, meats that are pumped full of antibiotics, growth hormones, steroids, etc. Don't forget the added acids & preservatives or pesticides & chemical poisons we consume in our food alone in addition to the poor air quality in many U.S. cities today. If you look at a typical U.S. diet in many cases it includes **a diet of food and beverages that is 60 – 70% acidic (toxic), is it any wonder why the majority of our population today is NOT healthy?**

If you've ever noticed someone who sweats profusely or has really bad body odor, that is usually the sign of a toxic person. In his book Toxemia Explained – The True Interpretation of the Cause of Disease, Dr. J. H. Tilden in his 50 years as an M.D. observed that "baby's breath is sweet and there is no foul odor in its perspiration since babies are designed to live off pure, raw human milk. Once switched to pasteurized milk, the baby's secretions become odorous & irritating with constipation often a result. Children who continue to drink lots of pasteurized cow's milk often have allergies and get sick more often." [7-2] If you've ever walked into a fraternity or sorority house on a Sunday morning after a keg party and lots of drinking, most everybody smells pretty putrid before hitting the shower and brushing their teeth. On the contrary I know of several vegetarians who don't use any deodorant. Their logic is their diet is so perfect (they excrete almost no smelly toxins) so they don't feel the need. The whole reason that pregnant woman get morning sickness is to expel any and all toxins from their womb creating a perfect, healthy environment for the fetus to develop and grow.

I'll never forget a focus group I attended last year in Los Angeles on fast foods. One of the large fast food chains paid us each $100 for an hour of our time to find out our perception of fast foods and eating habits. The focus group moderator went around the room asking questions until she stopped at this one poor lady. This lady had been laid off her job, her husband did not make that much money - he was only able to find part time work and they had 3 kids to feed. She described in detail how she would drive her kids to school every day and on the way she would get four (4) Wendy's Jr. bacon cheeseburgers for 99 cents each and four (4) large sodas. She would cut each of these bacon cheeseburgers in ½, so each child would get a meal for less than 50 cents each. The entire focus group had admitted earlier to seeing the documentaries "Food Inc." and "Super Size Me", so needless to say when we listened to this embarrassed lady describe how she had been feeding her kids for the past 2 years (every single day), we were flabbergasted. Nobody commented and the room fell silent while we listened to this poor lady tell her story and then sensing from the group that this was wrong, she literally broke down in tears crying: "I know this is so wrong what I'm doing to my kids. And I know it is not good for them as they often get sick, but I don't know what else I can possibly do to feed them when they are screaming that they are always hungry...". Inside I was crying for this lady and for her kids whom I had ever met. Now this true story is a little extreme, but is it any wonder why her kids are often sick if every single day, she's feeding her kids foods loaded with toxins? We all remember Morgan Spurlock (the director & star of "Super Size Me") who started puking in the McDonald's parking lot after a few days of a McDonald's only diet! If we put a consistent stream of toxins and poisons into our bodies each day, we WILL get sick, we WILL develop illnesses & disease, and for many of us we WILL most likely get cancer and die!

Let's sidestep the issue of flu-shots every year in this country (that is another discussion), but let me burst your bubble on the subject of viruses which people are afraid they are going to invade their bodies or think viruses are living creatures that attack us a certain time of the year. **Fact check: viruses are NOT living things**! Viruses are complicated assemblies of molecules, including proteins, nucleic acids, lipids, and carbohydrates, but on their own they can do nothing until they enter a living cell. Now ask yourself (whether or not you believe in flu-shots) when do most people in the U.S. catch a "virus" or catch a cold or flu? 99% of all the people I ask, can tell me exactly when the "cold & flu" season is. They all know that it is right after the Holidays (usually in January). It seems commonplace every single year around January where several members in my immediate family get sick (diarrhea, fever, exhaustion, sinus congestion, cough, etc.). Here's my theory and most nutritionists agree with me. It has very little to do with colder winter weather (although that can be a small factor). Everyone who catches the flu normally starts incubating this awful impending sickness around Halloween with unlimited candy treats (or cocktails & parties for the grown-ups). It continues with Thanksgiving where it's the tradition to overindulge ourselves with food, drinks, and extra deserts. Then during the month of

December there can be a dozen cocktail parties, work parties & end of the year celebrations with an abundance of toxic foods & lots of drinks. This ritual of over eating continues Christmas Eve, Christmas Day and culminates on New Year's Eve where wine, champagne, and an abundance of toxic foods once again tempt us. Many of us wake up January 1st starting off not with a gentle alkaline glass of wheat grass or cucumber juice (what would be best for your body), but a couple of glasses of coffee with some added sugar or artificial sweetener. To add to this recipe of disaster, most kids have a plethora of tests in December before their Holiday vacation, college students have final exams and papers, working people have end of the year deadlines, or business matters they must close out prior to December 31st, all of which create tremendous stress (more acid in your system). Add to this the reduced sleep schedule and for most people in a cold climate where daylight hours are very limited this also leads to people not exercising as much (limiting the effectiveness of your lymphatic system). To summarize for 3 straight months, we put more toxic foods & beverages into our body than any other time of the year, get less sleep, add more stress, and curtail our exercise schedule. By the time the Holidays are over, our bodies are a toxic cesspool leading to tens of millions of people catching a virus or flu every single January. After I figured this out, I consciously made the decision to hydrate during the Holiday season, super Alkalize, keep up a decent exercise schedule, and limit my portion sizes. As mentioned, while many of my family members get sick and catch the "flu" every January, I HAVE NOT BEEN SICK IN OVER 10 YEARS! I don't deprive myself of a nice Holiday meal, a small slice of pumpkin pie or a glass of wine or champagne on appropriate occasions, but I limit my portions and super-alkalize to counter the huge amount acids and toxins which are so prevalent during the Holidays. Think about this concept of toxins in your body carefully and you too can be one of the few who gets through this next Holiday season healthy & happy!

CHAPTER EIGHT (8):
The BEST Cure & the First Step...Juicing!

It should be crystal clear after reading the last few chapters how important proper alkalinity is to your well being, and there's no better way to way to alkalize your system than by juicing fresh, raw vegetables. We'll get into the specifics of the 7-Day "Alkalize & Energize" cleanse program in the next chapter, but here are just a few highlights of juicing.

By juicing, you get a maximum level of vitamins, minerals, and nutrients, and since you're drinking the juice in a 100% liquid form, the nutrients are quickly & easily absorbed. Eating (or drinking I should say) this liquid energy with nutrients your body needs, will give you an incredible amount of energy. By drinking all fluids, this also helps clean out your intestines and colon in comparison to people who eat a lot of red meat and other hard to digest foods, which can lead to colon cancer. Even the smallest food chunks & particles that don't get fully digested can get caught up in your colon, which if stretched out can easily extend over 4 feet in length. Often these particles fester, acidify, create gas and in the worst case can foster colon cancer. It is a total myth that overweight people have huge stomachs the size of basketballs. Your stomach should be about the size of your hand when closed to make a fist. Since the stomach muscle is elastic, it can stretch slightly when you pig out and eat way too much food at one sitting, but it may double in size in extreme cases. The truth about fat people you see waddling around the mall or Wal-Mart is that their intestines and colons have expanded over many years of overeating. Besides extra pounds of festering fecal matter lingering inside these organs, a host of other problems can happen including but not limited to: Irritable Bowel Syndrome, Spastic Colon, Crohn's Disease, Chronic Colitis, Leaky Gut Syndrome, Esophageal Reflux, Malabsorption Syndrome, Candida Albicans (yeast in the colon), and Chronic Fatigue Syndrome. Every nutritionist will agree and more medical doctors are starting to realize that juicing is the first step to excellent health. This has been in part due to new high-resolution blood imaging microscopes. Dr. Victor A. Marcial-Vega has some incredible footage, which he taped a patient whose blood is very typical of an American diet from a slightly acidic environment. The red blood cells are not very well rounded and in fact are stacked together like a roll of coins, and in other cases clumped together. There is also a lot of bacteria and fungus in the blood and the while blood cells you see do not look normal and are very sluggish. Dr. Vega then videotaped blood from the same patient a few days later and after the blood has become alkaline, the new video of the blood is astounding. The red blood cells are plump and perfectly round. They all have an electric charge on them so they are moving around, and not clumping together. There is very little bacteria, fungus or any other irregular cells in the video. On the video it also shows a big healthy white blood cell in action gobbling up some bacteria and other foreign particles. It is common sense that a person with an alkaline system and healthy blood cells will be able to carry much more oxygen, hence more energy! I encourage you to watch some of Dr. Vega's videos on YouTube of Alkaline blood vs. Acidic blood. The proof is right there in front of your eyes.

In addition to instant energy you'll get from the nutrients of the juice, ALL of the people we've worked with in addition to losing a few pounds lost 1 or more inches from their waist lines within the 1st 7 days! Loose fitting pants are a sign that you're starting to clean out your colon, but unlike an enema (which is also excellent for your health), this juicing cleanse will cleanse your entire digestive system (starting at the esophagus & ending at the rectum).

Jack LaLane discovered the powerful results of juicing when he was very young and opened up a juicing bar in his gym in 1936. Every 10 years or so he would do a stunt to prove that with his "juice" diet he was stronger and more fit than anyone else his age. One of the best publicity stunts I remember watching was when he was 70 years old, he had himself shackled and handcuffed yet still managed to tow a line of 70 boats over 1 mile through the middle of Long Beach harbor! While doing a TV appearance on his 95th birthday, he looked fitter than most 65 year olds (30 years younger) and he attributed all this to his juice diet & his daily exercise regimen.

Ronald shared his story with you about he had so much energy he turned into a "writing machine" cranking out books and screenplays like a factory. 2 of his books and 3 of his screenplays he finished up in one month! Looking back on some of my notes the first time I did a cleanse, in addition to feeling a "clarity" and peace of mind, my energy was very focused. Part of this might have been due to the fact that after the 3rd day of my cleanse I starved off all the candida (yeast) in my system, so my cravings for sugar & sweets went away completely. Since I wasn't eating any "inflammatory foods" (wheat, cereals, pastas, and flour products), my allergies improved noticeably. I had a tiny cut on my neck from shaving on the 5th day, which scabbed up and completely disappeared within a day! I never got any real hunger pangs after the 2nd day as I was constantly sipping lemon water and drinking my "Green" drink in between juicing. I was feeling better & better every single day and on the morning of the 6th day when I woke up I felt a little lethargic. There was no pain or discomfort at all and nothing like a hangover, but for some reason I felt a little tired for about an hour until going to the bathroom. That morning I excreted a large amount of waste and instantly (literally within seconds) felt energy like I've never felt before! A large chunk of toxins, etc. had just been cleared out of my body and when I did the weigh in I had dropped 3 pounds that day. The night of the 7th day happened to be a Sunday night and like most Sundays I was planning my busy week ahead. The problem (if you can call it that) was that I had so much energy I literally went for a 5-mile bike ride around my neighborhood at midnight. Normally I'd be sound asleep by 10 or 10:30pm since I'm an early riser, but that is the type of energy you can experience when you do the 7-Day "Alkalize & Energize" cleanse. I can't wait for you to get this same feeling you probably haven't felt since you were a little kid!

I could go on and on about the benefits of juicing as there are so many, but one of the comments almost all of the people we worked with make is how well they start sleeping. One older gentleman who always had trouble sleeping started getting 5 – 6 hours of totally uninterrupted sleep whereas before he was lucky to get 1 or 2 hours before he started tossing and turning. It's common sense that if you don't have a lot of extra sugars and caffeine in your body you will sleep better. Also since you haven't ingested pounds of crappy solid food all day and night, it also make sense that you are giving your entire digestive system a rest during the night. My next door neighbor complained of having stomach pains and lack of sleep last night (yesterday was Thanksgiving) and in the same sentence he went on and on about how much food he ate for several hours during all the Thanksgiving day festivities... is it really a surprise that he didn't get a restful sleep last night?

Another bonus of juicing and a point to really think about is that when you start juicing (whether for 7 days or if you continue for 90 days like Ronald did), you are shedding the many toxins & poisons that have built in your system. But you are also shedding DEAD CELLS! That's right... almost every cell in your body is replaced with new cells over time. Some cells are replaced in a few days, some a few months, and other are replaced in a few years. In theory you could have almost a completely NEW body in just 5 – 10 years, so why not make the decision to make it a brand new healthy one!

"If I had my way I'd make health catching
instead of disease."
- **Robert Ingersoll**

CHAPTER NINE (9): Ready? Instructions for the 7-Day "Alkalize & Energize" Cleanse!

The next big step that will change your life (it certainly changed the lives of both authors) is starting your 7-day "Alkalize & Energize" Cleanse. This is NOT a fast or a fad diet, as your body will be getting plenty of nutrients each day. If you follow this program exactly as described, you should not get any hunger pangs as you'll be drinking three (3) juice meals each day as well as a great deal of water and "Green drink". Green drink is found in health food stores and a small 10 – 16 oz. container will run about $20 - $30. It is a dry power consisting of natural green vegetables, algae, wheat grass, & herbs that will completely alkalize your body while giving you lasting fuel. Just pour the green drink powder it into a water bottle or container, and simply shake and you are drinking pure alkaline energy! Your food intake will be all-liquid for 7 days, as this will clean out your intestines and your colon to start getting you back towards perfect health.

We've already helped dozens of people get healthy again and with the release of this book, we're looking forward to help thousands more. As Wes Beavis mentions in his book Fuel – The Energy You Need to Succeed: "Distractions are enemy number one for anyone with a goal." [9-1] Here are a few quick steps to make sure you don't get distracted and to ensure that this 7-Day "Alkalize & Energize" cleanse changes your life in ways you cannot imagine!

1. Get HONEST with yourself about your ENERGY:
Do you have steady energy all day long, or do you feel groggy when you wake up in the morning? Do you feel exhausted after a hard day's work and plop down in front of the TV set for 2 or 3 hours? Do you sometimes put off an important task or responsibility and justify that "it can be done tomorrow"?

2. Do a simple pH test to check your body's ACIDITY:
You can get a general idea of your pH level by using some pH test strips at your local pharmacy. While not as accurate as a complete blood test, placing a small amount of saliva or urine on a pH test strip should confirm that your

body is acidic. The only people who may have a neutral ph (or a slightly alkaline pH) are people who have done this type of cleanse in the last few months, or vegetarians who are very strict about their diet and eat only organic & alkaline foods.

3. Do a BMI test to see if you are one of majority of people who are overweight or OBESE: There are plenty of charts & tables you can reference, or you can plug in your height & weight at this web-link from the National Institute of Health: www.nhlbisupport.com/bmi. If you are a few pounds overweight (or not well within the parameters) you need to take action immediately! Don't do the classic "denial" routine while looking in the mirror and keep telling yourself: "Oh, I'm only 5 – 10 lbs. overweight and feel fine". If you are in your 20s and are just 5 lbs. overweight, the time to take action is now! People (who don't prioritize their health) tend to slowly add extra weight each decade. The person who is just 5 lbs. overweight in their 20s could easily add 5 lbs. every few years to the point where they get to the golden retirement years they could easily be 20 – 30lbs. overweight. If you are in your 60s now or see anybody in their 60s, 70s, or 80s, take a look around and be honest with the obesity you see. One gentleman who we helped recently picked up a 25lb. dumbbell at the gym and realized he was lugging around that extra weight every day...that was great motivation for change! For the record, both authors are the same weight and have the same waist size that they had 20 years ago, so getting back to your "ideal healthy weight" is achievable for most people!

4. Even if you think you have lots of energy, and you're not overweight, take a long hard look and assess your current HEALTH:
Are you taking any prescriptions or over the counter drugs on a regular basis? Do you get sick once or twice a year (including a "cold" or "flu")? While this is common today, this does not have to be "normal".

5. Make a COMMITMENT with your spouse, partner, family member or friend. It can even be a co-worker, but make sure you tell someone that you are changing your

DO THESE THINGS OR YOU WILL DIE... 5 SECRETS

body and regaining your perfect health in the next 7 days. My company (Nemours Marketing) now offers coaching if you want to have us help you through this (our contact information is at the end of this book). The reason why it's imperative to tell someone that you're doing this 7 day cleanse is I've seen people go thought the first 3 or 4 days and get tempted with 1 simple cup of coffee (which is very acidic), or they see a large tub of Oreo Cookies & Cream ice cream in the freezer calling out to them in the middle of the night and they quit a few days early. Think about the end result in just 7 days and NOT about a short-term temptation. Having a friend or coach will help you during these 7 days. In the event you do get tempted, here is the best question to ask yourself: "Is it really worth the 2 minutes of pleasure (perceived pleasure actually) eating that chocolate fudge brownie most likely loaded with sugar, corn syrup, preservatives & additives?" A better question to ask is: "Isn't it more important to forgo that 2 minutes of a sweet tasting snack, so that I can start regaining my perfect health in 7 days for the rest of my life?"

6. Set your GOALS in WRITING: If weight loss is your main goal, it's imperative that you set a table with the date and your weight measurement for each day you do this cleanse. If you post this on the refrigerator or somewhere in the kitchen, other people in your house will see it and support your efforts. The people who did not mark their progress every single day in writing had a much tougher time sticking with the 7 day cleanse and often times did not get good results.

7. REMOVE all toxic foods from your sight for 7 days. You don't have to throw away all processed, sugar laden, boxed or frozen foods, but do your best to eat, dispose of them, or at least store them out of sight. The only food which should be on your kitchen counter, on the top shelf of your refrigerator, or on your sideboard is fresh vegetables.

8. STICK with the PLAN! People with the best intentions will call us during the 2nd or 3rd day and ask if they can have a glass of fresh squeezed orange juice or snack on a banana. The answer is absolutely NO as these fruits have

a lot of sugar. During the 7-Day "Alkalize & Energize" cleanse you must get all of the sugars out of your body which will kill any Candida (yeast) you probably have in your system and truly alkalize your body's pH balance. Other than a few exceptions, all of your food consumed in these 7 days should be liquid. In the Appendix of this book you'll find the Instruction Sheet for the 7-day Cleanse as well as a Frequently Asked Questions (FAQ) page.

The other most common question I get from people we're coaching is: "What do I do if in the middle of the 7-Day cleanse if I have a business meeting with a client or an important family gathering?" Don't let this fear keep you procrastinating the most important decision in your life! (If you think this is an overly dramatic statement, is there anything more important in your life than your health?). Don't let this be an excuse to keep putting off the 7-day cleanse! There is always a way to handle this. If you're meeting up with a client for coffee, have a green tea instead. If you have an important lunch meeting, drink water and have a salad with no dressing (squeeze some lemon juice on it instead or a sugar laden salad dressing). If you have a family gathering, snack on some carrots & celery while drinking lots of water and politely tell them you are not that hungry. Having a green tea, a salad, or some raw veggies will stick keep you on track for these 7 days.

Wrapping up this chapter, I'd like to point out two (2) pitfalls which both authors fell into on one of their many cleanses they have done as "control experiments":

1. Ronald was doing the cleanse and after 3 – 4 days he figured that if he juiced only once a day he would limit his caloric intake and lose weight even faster...WRONG. For two days during one of Ronald's cleanses, Ronald stopped losing any weight as his body went into "starvation mode" meaning that his body sensed that he was not getting enough nutrients and held onto all body fat to coincide with the lack of nutrition he was getting.

2. I was doing an annual cleanse and one time I lost exactly 20 lbs. in 7 days dropping from 166 down to 146.

After day 7, I decided to run a fast 4-mile run (not a walk or slow jog as we recommend), and then decided to go to the gym for an upper body workout including several sets of curls. Before stopping the cleanse, I wanted to see if I would lose another 2- 3 lbs. (as I previously had every day), but I actually gained 1.4 lbs.! This was because when doing extreme exercise such as wind sprints, or working out with heavy weights, your muscles produce massive amounts of lactic acid. The extra acid in your body sends a signal to your cells to stop dumping fat, and instead you retain body fat to protect all of your organs. During the 7-day cleanse make sure you juice three (3) nutritious meals a day and avoid extreme or intense exercise which might create more acid in your system. What is OK, and recommended is walking, an easy bike ride, rollerblading, a relaxing yoga session, deep breathing & stretching exercises.

When you're ready to start your 7-Day "Alkalize & Energize" cleanse, make sure you look at the Information Sheet and the FAQ page in the Appendix. After you're done please call or write us, as we'd love to hear about your own success story back to perfect health!

"Sickness is the vengeance of nature
for the violation of her laws."
- Charles Simmons

CHAPTER TEN (10):
Another Antacid Commercial!

30 years ago, you might have seen an occasional Alka-Seltzer ad, but today if you watch television or read any magazines, you're going to see a plethora of antacid drug ads due to our "SAD" American diet. (SAD stands for "Standard American Diet"). Due to the abundance of acidic foods in today's diets, the single drug segment (antacid medications) has grown to billions of dollars of revenues in the U.S. alone! Doctors now prescribe antacid medications by the ton in this country, not only due to our highly acidic diet, but also because Americans are generally overweight, love to eat large meals & deserts, and prefer fatty foods and things like sodas, coffee, alcohol, chocolate, sweets, spicy foods, etc. all of which worsen acid-reflux. Some pharmaceutical companies are now sending FREE antacid sample pills in the mail (I got several Prilosec pills) in my mailbox just last week! Powerful acid blockers are available over the counter now that a few years ago were only available by prescription. Physicians prescribe many different types of antacids because their patients crave them (after seeing the millions of advertisements including in the doctor's waiting room) and there are no "perceived" down sides. These antacid medications including PPIs (proton pump inhibitors) and other acid blockers can create dozens of health risks and side effects. If you don't believe me, just read the back page of any anti-acid magazine ad or try to listen to the list of side effects that are rattled off in the last 3 seconds of a 30 second television ad. These side effects of different prescriptions can include: dizziness, nausea, vomiting, blurred vision, loss of breath, depression, even death! I'm not joking and if you're like me, you probably can't understand a single word the announcer says due to how ridiculously fast those disclaimers of health risks are read off! Despite the side effects, antacids have become so mainstream that according to WebMD, generic Prilosec (omeprazole), one single antacid drug now is issued for 53.4 million annual prescriptions! Prilosec is only one (1) single drug and that does not include any competitive antacid drugs or over the counter sales!

After reading the 1st few chapters, it should be obvious that increased acids in your diet (and in most of your body now) could be a huge problem. I'm not suggesting that you immediately stop taking antacid pills (either over the counter) or those prescriptions if you need them without consulting your doctor, but why not be brutally HONEST with yourself? Is it possible that with the quantity and quality of food and beverages in your diet, you might be creating some of this extra acid in your system? For some of you, I would bet $100 the answer is yes. It's common sense then, NOT to keep putting a "band-aid" on these symptoms, but it's time to get to the root cause of this excess acid and start eliminating it (or at least reducing it) from your diet! Several of the 50 folks we've now worked with (and who started with our 7-Day "Alkalize & Energize" cleanse) have totally eliminated the need to take ANY antacid medications! Why not you? Or you could keep watching television commercials the rest of your life and just keep "taking a pill"? The choice is yours.

"Was the government to prescribe to us
our medicine and diet,
our bodies would be in such keeping
as our souls are now."
- Thomas Jefferson

<u>CHAPTER ELEVEN (11)</u>: "Common" vs. Normal

Society's perception of health is much different today than it was just 30 years ago. This past year when I went home for Christmas, my mother and other family members commented how I was "too skinny". Is that really true or is that a perception based upon what is "common" in today's population? Just because the majority of the U.S. population is now slightly overweight or obese, that does not make me too skinny or unhealthy. In the U.S. today, it's "common" that at least ½ of a typical 5th grade classroom may be overweight, but that does not mean it's normal. Both authors were commenting that it's normal that most of our friends in their 30s or 40s have added at least 10 – 20 lbs. over their high school weight. In fact, both authors at the time of publishing weigh their exact high school weight. This is certainly uncommon, but this should not be abnormal. It is very "common" to see people in their 60s or 70s who now that have arthritis, or spinal stenosis. It is now "common" to hear about people in their 30s or 40s who are already taking prescriptions every day for high blood pressure or high cholesterol levels. This may be more & more common, but this is NOT normal! When all schools used to have mandatory physical education classes (many have been eliminated due to school budget cuts) and before kids had access to the internet, hundreds of cable channels, and thousands of video games, it was normal for kids to get lots of daily exercise. Now it's uncommon that kids get that kind of exercise (hence the child obesity epidemic in this country). Another marker is the common portions of today's food before the "Super Size" or "Super Big Gulp" mentality, which has become normal. How about the new "Triple Whopper" with cheese from Burger King which boats over 1,200 calories and 87 grams of fat or Wendy's Baconator Double which boast almost 1,000 calories and plenty of meat? More and more restaurants, hotels, theme parks, convenience stores, etc. push the larger sizes to fuel their profits. People don't think twice about today's "common" sizes, but maybe you'll reconsider what is normal after looking at the following chart. The % increase for all these different foods and beverages is frightening. No wonder the U.S. is ranked as the "most obese" country in the world.

ITEM	SIZE & CALORIES: 30 YEARS AGO	SIZE & CALORIES: TODAY	% SIZE INCREASE
Soda	8 oz. Coca-Cola bottle (26 grams of sugar)	40 oz. Big Gulp (130 grams of sugar)	500%
Coffee	8 oz. cup (40 calories)	16 oz. cup (300 – 400 calories)	200%
Bagel	3" in diameter (140 Calories)	Up to 6" in diameter (350 calories)	200%
Cheeseburger	single patty (1.6 oz.)	single patty (4 oz. = ¼ lb.)	250%
Popcorn served at Movie theaters	Medium bag 5 cups (up to 300 calories)	Medium tub 20 cups (up to 1,200 calories)	400%
Empty restaurant plate (no food)	9 inches	12 inches	133%
Empty restaurant cup (no fluid)	8 – 10 oz.	16 oz.	200%

One important concept to understand for perfect health is the more "excess" food you put into your system, the more you are overloading and "taxing" the systems in your body including your stomach, entire digestive system, lymphatic system, etc. In every medical & scientific study I've reviewed, the subjects (both humans and animals) which ate smaller food portions & quantities have been the healthiest and have always lived the longest. On the television program Nova Science Now, the scientists and medical experts concluded that a calorie restrictive diet helped ALL the animals tested live longer. [11-1]

Of course this does not mean to starve yourself. This proven theory is AFTER you've provided your body with the necessary calories and nutrients. This also applies to the 7-day juicing you do to "energize and alkalize" your system. Do NOT try and drink 2 or 3 huge glasses of vegetable juice at one time as you will be taxing your system and creating expensive urine. One (1) 16 – 20 oz. glass of juice has enough nutrients for a full meal. Drinking an excess amount of alkaline wheat grass or vegetable juice (no matter how good it is for you) will be counterproductive. The specific instructions on how to do the 7-Day "Alkalize & Energize" juice program are in the Appendix at the end of the book. It has worked amazing for both authors and dozens of other people we've worked with the past few years. Speaking of "alkalizing" your system, the following is an extensive list of "common" ailments, sicknesses, and diseases, which may be reduced, eliminated, or alleviated with an alkaline diet (along with exercise described in detail in section IV). It was not normal 30 – 40 years ago for so many people in the U.S. population to have cancer and many other diseases and it is a national tragedy that these diseases and illnesses have become "normal". Once again, there is no 100% guarantee your illness or disease can be cured by alkalizing your system, but many other people have weaned their way off some or all of their prescription drugs with an alkaline diet, lost weight, and feel better then they ever have before, so if you have any of these health issues listed below, why not try to get back to perfect health? You have nothing to lose except for a few extra pounds!
(listed in alphabetical order)

ADD (Attention Deficit Disorder)
ADHD (Attention Deficit/Hyperactivity Disorder)
ACE (Adverse Childhood Experiences)
ALS (Amyotrophic Lateral Sclerosis)
Alzheimer's Disease
Antibiotic and Antimicrobial Resistance
Aortic Aneurysm

Arthritis (several types including Osteoarthritis &
Rheumatoid Arthritis)
Asthma
Abdominal Aortic Aneurysm
Abdominal Pain
Abnormal Heart Rhythms (Heart Rhythm Disorders)
Abnormal Liver Enzymes
Accumulation of Fluid in the Abdominal Cavity (Ascites)
Aches, Pain, Fever
Acid Reflux (Heartburn & Gastroesophageal Reflux)
Acne (& Acne Rosacea)
Acquired Bronchiectasis
Athlete's Foot
Bleeding Disorders
Blood Cancers
Blood Disorders
Bone Health (including bone density loss)
Bronchitis
BV (Bacterial Vaginosis)
Cancer (including: Cervical, Colon, Gynecologic Cancers,
Hematologic Cancers, Prostate Cancers)
Candida Infection (Candidiasis)
Capillaria Infection (Capillariasis)
Cardiovascular Health
CFS (Chronic Fatigue Syndrome)
Chest Cold (Bronchitis)
Childhood Diseases (many types)
Childhood Overweight and Obesity
Chlamydia Pneumonia Infection
Cholesterol Level Elevation
Chronic Constipation
Common Cold
COPD (Chronic Obstructive Pulmonary Disease)
Crohn's Disease
Diabetes (especially Type II)
Diarrhea
Diphtheria (Corynebacterium Diphtheria Infection)
Depression & Mood Swings
DVT (Deep Vein Thrombosis)
Ear Infection (Otitis Media)
Elephantiasis (Lymphatic Filariasis)
Epilepsy
Ergonomic and Musculoskeletal Disorders

Fibromyalgia
Filariasis (Lymphatic)
Flu (many different kinds including Seasonal & Influenza)
Food-Related Diseases (many types)
Gonorrhea
Gout (& Gout related complications)
Healthcare Associated Infections (almost all infections)
Heart Disease (many different types of cardiovascular diseases)
High Blood Pressure
HPS (Hantavirus Pulmonary Syndrome)
Hypertension
IBD (Inflammatory Bowel Disease)
Impetigo
Infertility
Iron Deficiency (Anemia)
Liver Disease (usually directly created by acids)
Lymphatic Filariasis
LCMV (Lymphocytic Choriomeningitis)
Lymphoma
Micronutrient Malnutrition
Migraine Headaches
Nutrition Diseases (multiple types)
OA (Osteoarthritis)
Obesity and Overweight Illnesses
Osteoporosis
PAD (Peripheral Arterial Disease)
Parasitic Diseases (multiple types)
Pneumonia (many different types)
Pulmonary Hypertension
Scabies
Seasonal Flu (many different types of flu)
Shingles (Varicella Zoster Virus)
Sinus Infection (many types of Sinusitis)
Skin Infections (& chronic scabs)
Sleep Apnea (& many other Sleep Disorders)
Sore Mouth Infection (Orf Virus)
Sore Throat (& Strep Throat infections)
Stomach Flu (Viral Gastroenteritis)
Stomach Expansion (requiring new Lap Band procedures)
Streptococcus pneumonia Infection
Stress (including occupational)

Stroke
Thrombophilia (Clotting Disorders)
Toxin Sickness (usually created by acids in system)
Trachoma Infection
Ulcerative Colitis (Inflammatory Bowel Disease)
Vaginal Yeast Infection
Vertigo (dysfunction of the Vestibular System)
Vision Impairment
Weight Gain problems

"The patient should be made to understand that he or
she must take charge of his own life.
Don't take your body to the doctor
as if he were a repair shop."
- **Quentin Regestein**

CHAPTER TWELVE (12):
The Problem With Diets... Most Don't Work!

Nobody (including myself) at Nemours Marketing is sponsored by, or has ANY ties with any supplement, nutrition, drug, or diet companies. While this book mentions a few products that may work for you, 95% of what is recommended are fresh, live foods (mostly vegetables, fruits, nuts, sprouts, etc.) that you can buy at your local grocery store or farmer's market. Doing research for this book, I read over 100 books on nutrition, exercise, general health, biology, anatomy, chemistry, diet, and general medicine. It seemed like almost every other new book on the market was a "Diet" book! Many people try to capitalize on the desperation of overweight, unhealthy people while getting their share of the billion-dollar diet industry that has spawned thousands of diet books many of them contradicting each other. A few (though not all) of these Diet book authors also try to sell you on the "book of the month", get you hooked on expensive diet supplements, push expensive concoctions, or promote costly memberships, etc. I will leave those options up to you, but honestly all the healthy foods you'll be eating can be purchased for very little money going back to the basic vegetables, salads, fruits, nuts, and sprouts, etc. that should make up the bulk of your diet. Important: ANY diet that does not focus on alkalinity (promoting mostly vegetables & salads) while also talking about some form of exercise is a SCAM. This doesn't mean you can't eat fish or occasionally eat chicken, limited red meats, dairy, etc. but MOST (at least 80%) of your food consumed should be alkaline & water-rich foods.

Statistics prove over and over again that most (over 50%) of all diets don't get lasting results. The problem with most diets is that the dieter gets hungry, cranky, fatigued, and often gets deprived of nutrition and calories their body needs. The 1st 3 letters of diet read D-I-E... that should give you a clue that your body is being deprived! You know how the story of most diets ends. After a few weeks or months, most dieters go on a "binge" and gain back most of the extra weight they started with over time. One friend (who I thought was very healthy conscious) and did in fact lose 60 lbs., later gained over half of that weight back over the Holidays by what he calls "sport eating". He eats as much as he wants when he wants, and equates the challenge to a "sport". To me this is tragic if you really know what is good for your body. Once you understand the negative effects of processed & acidic foods (you hopefully will by the end of this 1st section), you will want to change over to the healthy "lifestyle" which one again should be comprised of 80% live, alkaline, all natural water-rich foods.

After you give yourself the gift of the 7-Day "Alkalize & Energize" cleanse, your mindset will most likely change and you will see food as nutritious energy. This is NOT a diet or a fast, as you are getting a good amount of calories, and lots of nutrition (including vitamins & minerals) in the form of alkaline vegetable juices. It is rather a gentle cleanse that produced amazing results for over 50 people we worked with prior to the book's release. As mentioned, contributing author Ronald Farnham lost 60 lbs. of fat & toxins in just 90 days while his energy level went through the roof so much that he hardly sleeps right now and in less than 1 year has written 3 other books and ½ a dozen film screenplays! The 7-day program will really change your life, but unlike a DIET, you won't starve or deprive yourself. You should see amazing results and be able to transition from there into a healthy lifestyle you'll be able to maintain like my friend Rick who's kept off the 100+ lbs he lost for over 2 years now and looks younger & healthier than he did 5 years ago! Most importantly since he is eating an 80% alkaline diet, he has more energy and feels better than every before! In the next chapter, we'll cover how to ensure LASTING SUCCESS with your new alkaline eating habits and lifestyle, so keep reading!

CHAPTER THIRTEEN (13):
LASTING Success with an Alkaline ~~Diet~~ Lifestyle

It's My Life! author Richard Walker monitored his body fat changes for 4 months and shares an important lesson when he remarked: "I found the more strict I became with my diet and the more rigorous my workouts became (at one point doubling the daily workout to twice daily), the less results I achieved." [13-1]. The bottom line is to remember that you should NOT be dieting, depriving, or starving yourself in any way. After you cleanse and balance out your body's pH level, you can eat different foods as long as you approach your new lifestyle with common sense incorporating an 80% alkaline diet and consuming the same (or less) amount of calories that you burn each day. The reason I crossed out the word DIET is looking at the 1st three letters D I E, it is a symbolic, negative reminder that Diets can often deprive ourselves until we die. The proper definition of DIE from the Merriam-Webster dictionary is "to pass from physical life (expire) or "to pass out of existence (cease)". I'm not calling this program a diet, because it starts with a life changing "alkalizing & energizing" cleanse and continues with a healthy balanced lifestyle. What good is a fad diet if 6 months later, you gain part (or all) of the weight back? What good is the effort if a year later, you go back to a place where you don't have the same high level of energy which comes from being less toxic & completely healthy? One of my mentors Tony Robbins captured my attention on the subject of health because he only looks at long-tem lasting results. You wouldn't study a wealthy millionaire if 5 years later he or she lost all of their money, so why would you listen to anyone (including a Medical Doctor who may have limited nutritional training) if that doctor, author, or speaker gained part of their weight back or lived an unhealthy lifestyle? I find it humorous in those cases where people will often go visit their doctor who happens to be 30 pounds overweight and taking 2 – 3 prescription drugs and this is the expert you are taking advice from to lose weight and get healthy?! I'm now coaching people (on-line, via telephone, and in person), and morally have the responsibility to live what I am preaching. While I might now be considered "middle age", most people say I look much younger than my real age and I am well within my BMI range weighing under 165 lbs. on a 6-foot frame. That is less than my high school weight several decades ago! Most importantly I have more energy than ever before and is able to run just as far and lift heavier weights than I could decades ago while on the high school football team! I don't want to brag, but I do wanted to share an incredible story, which happened last month. I was on a film set and a friend Gene Wallace (whom I had not seen for about 2 years) came up to me and said: "Wow... Scott, you look great! You look 5 or 10 years younger that the last time I saw you!" You too can get those complements when you cleanse your system out, exercise every day and hydrate your entire body like we'll cover in section III.

In short, there's a reason why you should believe what you are reading in this book. The authors (myself and contributing author Ronald) both have a healthy lifestyle that has been working long-term! It's not our job to call out other authors, medical doctors (neither of us have medical degrees), but it is common sense to look at any diet or prescribed lifestyle and research the long-term results! Many of you reading this book might have tried a diet one time and it either didn't work or years later you slipped back to where you started in terms or health, weight, or energy. The results of failed diets are consistent with most reports showing that approximately 80% of people who go on a diet fail long-term (meaning they gain part or all of the weight back), or they slip back into an acid diet or an unhealthy lifestyle. Estelle Toby Goldstein, M.D. who changed her lifestyle in a dramatic way has seen studies that show up to 95% of people show go on a diet have gained weight back!" It might be worth reading Dr. Goldstein's book This is Not a Diet Book, as she is one of the few doctors today who does not recommend any diet, surgery, or prescriptions. The reason patients listen to Dr. Goldstein is because she has PROVEN results with her patients and also with herself. Besides losing well over 100 lbs., here is Dr. Goldstein's powerful results in her own words: "Today I weigh less than half of what I did then — only slightly over two years ago. My blood pressure was sky high — now it is normal. My blood sugar was dangerously diabetic — now it is normal. My triglycerides were so high, I was a walking stroke-risk — now they are normal." [13-2] You can read more about Dr. Goldstein at her website: www.estelletobygoldstein.com

An important thing for YOU to do after your 7-Day "Alkalize & Energize" cleanse is to note the change in energy, health & vitality. I strongly encourage you to make notes or write a journal entry how you feel before and after. After you transition from the 7 days (of juicing only alkaline vegetables) and transition to a healthy balanced lifestyle (in which 80% of all your food and drink is alkaline and you limit any acidic or processed food to no more than 20%), you must program your mind why you want to stay healthy. I, myself have made incredible health a MUST, and not a SHOULD. There are many great psychological tools you can use to get leverage on living a healthy lifestyle, one of which is a new smart phone application where you can take a picture of yourself and then press a button to make your face or your whole body "fat". Seeing a visual like that is very powerful and is an excellent tool to remind you that a healthy lifestyle should be a MUST for you also! If you need more leverage to help you lose weight, another great way to get leverage on yourself to follow though is to pick up a 20 lb. dumbbell the next time you are in the gym. If you are just 20 lbs. overweight, imagine carrying that heavy dumbbell around every single day! If you never go to the gym, the next time you're at the grocery store, pick up a gallon of milk, which weighs just over 9 lbs. Now try carrying two (2) of these gallon milk jugs around the store for just a few minutes. That is what it would feel like to be just 18 lbs. overweight. Imagine carrying around all this extra weight every single day!

There are times like when I visited a friend's film set last week where after lunch I thought for a minute that I also wanted a big slice of cherry cheese cake that everyone else seemed to be enjoying (and they probably were for the 2 – 3 minutes while they were eating their sweet treat desert). However, I have now conditioned my mind to look at the long-term pleasure of NOT putting that store bought processed calorie & sugar laden, artery clogging, fattening cheese cake into my body as I know all the extra sugar and dairy will make me sluggish the rest of the afternoon. I used to be a Mountain Dew™ addict. At one point, I would drink 2 – 3 liters a day especially at night when all the extra caffeine & sugar would give me a boost while I was working long hours in my office sometimes until 1 or 2am. Over a long period of time, I didn't notice that people started calling me Niki's older brother (my sister Niki is 8 years older than me!). My hair was thinning, I was stressed a lot, and although not really overweight I had two large "love handles" that I could never, ever get rid of no matter how many sit-ups I did. FYI...the love handles (which vex so many people) completely went away after I alkalized! After the 1st time I juiced and got back to my body's perfect health, I vowed to appreciate and keep the incredible health that I reclaimed. To this day (it has been over 6 years), I have lived this healthy lifestyle and over 80% of all the food and drink I put in my body is alkaline, organic, alive, and healthy. The key to lasting results is mental. You need to condition your psychology that this great health, energy, and vitality is much more important that 2 or 3 minutes of "perceived" pleasure based upon the signals your taste buds send to your brain for that short time. When I go home for the Holidays with family, I'll enjoy the food that my mother and stepmother prepare and celebrate with everyone else in the family. I might even enjoy an occasional Coke or glass of red wine and at a pizza party where I may have one or two slices of vegetarian pizza, but my overall lifestyle is healthy and balanced. I have no urge to pig out on Holiday sweets or load up on an extra portion of red meat.

An excellent guide that I've posted in my kitchen is the "Food Thoughts for Healthy Living... 80% Alkaline / 20% Acid" poster which you can find in Dr. Baroody's book titled Alkalize or Die which is a must read. With this guide posted on your refrigerator, a healthy mind set (and some coaching or support initially from whoever you choose, even if it is a good friend or family member), you can live a long healthy, happy life. The alternative is not pretty and hence the reason why I came up with the title of this book: Do These Things or You Will Die! Here's some "food for thought" (excuse the pun) if you still don't feel compelled to live a healthy lifestyle yourself. If you have kids, nieces or nephews of any friends with kids carefully ponder this statistic from a recent USA Today article: "Diabetes and pre-diabetes have skyrocketed among the nation's young people, jumping from 9% of the adolescent population in 2000 to 23% in 2008" [13-3]. In addition, new reports in 2012 are showing child and teen obesity rates in the United States now reaching as high as 33%! If you don't take the information in this book seriously and take ACTION NOW, you could be part of this startling statistic recently reported from HealthDay: "The number of obese people in the United States will increase from 99 million in 2008 to 164 million by 2030" [13-4]. That means half our country could be obese and afflicted with all the disease, sickness, afflictions, and potential for cancer unless we educate people about this growing epidemic!

I wish you all the best success with the first step of changing your health in 7 days and hope you transition this into a long lasting, healthy lifestyle. Once again, please drop me a note with your success. I look forward to hearing about your own success story!

⇔ SUBSTITUTE: The next time you're hungry or just plain out of energy, don't just grab any pre-packaged snack or sweet treat. Always make sure to have REAL foods around like fresh fruit, or delicious home made Trail-Mix made with almonds, cashews, raisins, and coconut. You will satisfy your hunger while doing your body some good.

SECTION II:
OXYGENATE

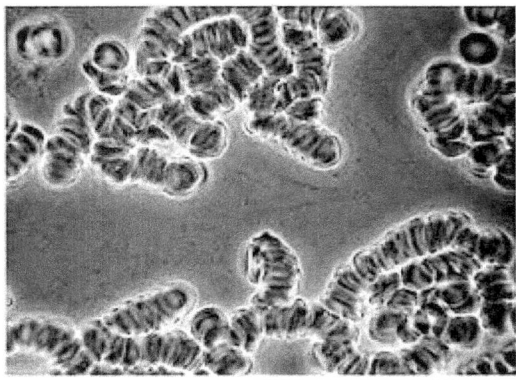

"Acidic" blood where the red blood cells are clumped together reducing the effective transport of oxygen. The dark spots are candida (yeast), bacteria, and fungus developing in this toxic environment.
(Photo courtesy of NaturalFatLoss.com)

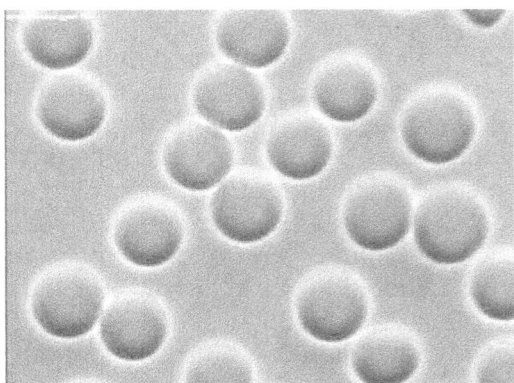

An "alkaline" environment. The red blood cells are perfectly round & plump. The "alkaline electric" charge outside cell helps them move rapidly to carry lots of oxygen without sticking to each other.
Notice also how clean the blood is!
(Photo courtesy of NaturalFatLoss.com)

CHAPTER FOURTEEN (14): TAKE THE 0^2 TEST

Before moving to the next chapter on how important oxygen is, it's critical to understand that if your body does not get enough oxygen, you could get permanent brain damage in just 3 minutes and possibly die a few minutes later without this critical element!

There are many factors that determine your lung capacity including height, weight, sex, age, etc. but the average lung capacity is between 4 – 6 liters. There are two extremes you've probably noticed in terms of lung capacity: 1) an older person (usually a smoker) who gets almost NO exercise and is hooked up to an oxygen tank and 2) any athlete, aerobics instructor, or yoga guru who most likely has more than a 6 liter capacity. A person who lives in the mile high city of Denver will normally have a higher lung capacity than a person living below sea level in New Orleans, so altitude plays a factor as well.

As sad as it sounds, I've met some sedentary people who can't take a deep breath in, hold their breath, and then exhale (a complete breath cycle) for more than 15 seconds. Stop reading right now and do this quick test with a stopwatch or timer. You should NOT strain or push yourself in any way, but with the timer going breath in through your nose.... hold as long as you comfortably can.... and slowly exhale through your mouth. If you are an athlete, you should be able to exceed 30 seconds. If you are a walker or someone who does moderate exercise every day you should be able to last 15 – 20 seconds. If you can't make this simple exercise last at least 12 seconds, please be HONEST with yourself. If you're at all worried about your lung capacity, ask yourself a few simple questions:

1) When you walk up just 1 flight of stairs, do you feel slightly winded?

2) If you get out of bed too quickly in the morning, do you ever get dizzy?

3) Is it difficult for you to walk short distances (perhaps just a ½ mile)?

If you answered YES to any of the above questions, ask yourself the question how often you are exercising? Maybe NOW is a good time to start! If you are still worried, the next time you see your doctor, he or she can do a simple Lung Function Test (also called a Pulmonary Function Test).

"When it comes to eating right & exercising,
there is no 'I'll start tomorrow.' Tomorrow is disease!"
- V.L. Allineare

CHAPTER FIFTEEN (15): OXYGEN...
The Key to Healthy Cells and an Energetic Life

Nobel Prize winner Dr. Otto Warburg made some amazing discoveries in 1931 on the importance of oxygen being one of the keys to healthy cells. His discoveries opened up new ways in the fields of cellular metabolism and cellular respiration. Dr. Warburg demonstrated time & time again that cancerous cells live and develop in the absence of oxygen. On the contrary, he also found it was almost impossible for cancer to thrive (let alone exist) in a fully oxygenated cell. Nobel Prize honoree Dr. Alexis Carrel started an experiment on January 17, 1912 where he placed tissue cultured from an embryonic chicken heart in a stoppered Pyrex flask. He maintained the living culture for over 20 years with regular supplies of nutrients including oxygen, which was almost twice a chicken's normal lifespan of 11 years! This wildly successful experiment conducted at the Rockefeller Institute for Medical Research was finally terminated as he had proved the importance of fully oxygenated cells that could help cells live almost indefinitely! Dr. Carrel's work proved time and time again that fully oxygenated cells help maintain perfect health.

Dr. Morris F. Keller is the author of an informative book titled: Setting Yourself Apart from the Seeds of Cancer and explains: "Yeast infections, such as candida albicans occur most frequently in an oxygen poor environment in the body. Currently, I would say that, we have an epidemic of common yeast infections in our modern society. Yeast cells produce large amounts of acetaldehyde - which cause cellular damage, interfere with intestinal absorption and disrupt white and red blood cell functions. Increasing O^2 levels in our body and eliminating commercial yeast and sugary foods from our diets will lessen this problem." [15-1]

Luckily there is much more awareness about the importance of oxygen and all the extraordinary health benefits. In addition to "Oxygen Bars" opening up in different cities where people for a few dollars can inhale fresh oxygen to get energized, there are now companies offering oxygen "masks" where you can infuse fresh oxygen to your skin. These masks pump fresh oxygen into your pores and boost your skin's elasticity, which gives your skin a plumper, healthier look. The oxygen can make wrinkles, redness, scales, or other forms of skin irritation less noticeable for several days after treatment. Oxygen can also minimize any acne or skin irritations teenagers often get. After seeing the amazing results on some friends who use the Bliss™ brand oxygen mask, I wanted to share this tip in case any of you want to look into this for great youthful skin. Since the epidermis (your skin) is the largest human organ in your body, starting to oxygenate the largest organ in your body can't hurt!

Getting back to the more traditional way of getting oxygen into your cells, you've have probably heard your parents say a thousand times when you were younger to "go outside and get some exercise". Any legitimate doctor will agree that diet & exercise are two keys to better health and a longer life, yet ironically many U.S. doctors are not that healthy. Instead of boring you with dozens of other specific references of medical experiments proving the importance of oxygenating cells to maintain perfect health in the next chapter, we'll look at the some people who are pumping fresh oxygen into their cells daily and living perfect health!

"A healthy body and soul come from an
unencumbered mind and body."
- Ymber Delecto

CHAPTER SIXTEEN (16):
A Valuable Lesson from Athletes

On an energy level scale from 1 to 10, zero (0) would be the bottom of the scale where you are getting NO new oxygen pumped through your system as your lungs have stopped working and you're DEAD! Level 10 would be someone in perfect health who just finished a moderate run, or an aerobics or yoga class where you have enabled your lungs to pump fresh oxygen throughout your system and removed the waste product carbon dioxide. Most people who don't get regular physical activity (specifically aerobic activity) go through life at a 5 or 6 energy level. Many people working for long hours at their computer or trapped in a cubicle for 3 – 4 straight hours with no fresh oxygen, very little body movement, and no deep breathing would represent an energy level 2 or 3. It's common sense that after a nice jog, a brisk 15-minute walk, or any other kind of aerobic exercise you will be more alert, have more energy, and simply feel better. In addition to gaining more energy, oxygenating your system is one of the most important keys to perfect health and reducing your chance for serious illness, disease, or cancer. Back tracking a little, your body takes about 20,000 breaths each day. With the help of your lungs, air is taken in through your nose, filtered and sent into the many different branches in your lungs called bronchioles ending up in grape-like sacs called alveoli, which are surrounded by capillaries. It is here that oxygen gets separated and then taken into the blood stream where oxygenated blood cells get transported to other cells all around your body. The same time carbon dioxide transfers from your bloodstream back into the alveoli where is then exhaled out of the body. The great news is that with regular breathing exercises, you can make your lungs stronger and more efficient. In just a few weeks time, you can increase the amount of oxygen your body takes in and actually increase the number and efficiency of capillaries you have around your air sacs.

On a BeWellBuzz.com podcast, cancer expert and author of Cancer – Step Outside the Cure shared a shocking World Health Organization statistic that 41% of Americans will be diagnosed with cancer in their lifetimes! [16-1]. Of course much of this has to do with increased acids and toxicity from the poor diet here in the U.S. Several studies reveal that professional athletes are up to seven (7) times less likely to get cancer than the average person due partly to their exercise routine and the fact they are fully oxygenating their system. One of my good friends Bruce Ellington (who we worked with and had incredible results last year in his 7-Day "Alkalize & Energize" cleanse) used to be an Olympic athlete. He was one of the best high jumpers in the country and started playing sports at an early age continuing through high school and college (University of Kansas) until he was inside the LA Coliseum wearing red, white, and blue for the opening of the 1984 Olympics. Marching in the company of teammates Carl Lewis, Michael Jordan, Greg Louganis, and Marylou Retton is certainly every kid's dream! Bruce's story is interesting as he grew up in the 60's and 70s with both his parents working, so he had to fend for himself in the kitchen. Not knowing any better, Bruce's daily breakfast consisted of Coke, bacon, and Frosted Flakes cereal while lunch at school was usually a few slices of pepperoni pizza, French fries, washed down with lots of cherry Kool-Aid. Dinner was either a burger or macaroni & cheese followed by a bowl or two of ice cream and some more soda. (Basically his diet consisted of corn syrup, sugar, enriched wheat flour, fat & carcinogens, red meat, and more sugar). I was absolutely horrified when he shared this with me! Bruce did pay the price though as he occasionally got sick and had constant allergies growing up. At the height of his "toxic dumping" (the acidic processed food he fueled his body with), Bruce got a bad case of mono-nucleosis, and later tonsillitis. Luckily he never became obese and by some miracle never got diabetes. The reason Bruce didn't gain a lot of weight is he was burning all the calories he was consuming with his intense athletic regimens and workouts. In the previous chapter you learned how important oxygen is to good health and when serious athletes like Bruce are super-oxygenating their system every single day, this is a large factor in maintaining good health. My best friend in elementary school (Fritz Collister) had a similar diet when he was growing up including lots of sweets and candies, but he was not athletic at all. Sadly Fritz died very young in his 20s and I often wonder if this poor nutrition and lack of exercise played a role in his demise. There is a second reason athletes are so energetic and healthy is that through constant muscle movement they are stimulating their lymphatic system, which clears out toxins and waste from their bodies. Bruce wonders to this day how great an athlete he might have been if he had combined his workout rituals and training with a good diet. You'll learn more about the critical lymphatic system in chapter 18. But fully oxygenating your body is so powerful, in my opinion it's the main reason why most serious athletes:

1) have an abundance of energy

2) get a restful sleep

3) have the ability to recover from injuries so quickly

4) have glowing skin

5) have a much higher endurance for physical activity

6) can in many cases tolerate a poor diet (although I would NOT recommend testing this)

If you know any serious athlete (people training seriously at least 6 days a week) whether at the high school, collegiate, professional, or Olympic levels you'll agree with these observations. People who are serious and dedicated yoga enthusiasts (also super-oxygenating their bodies) have the same characteristics. Now I don't condone Bruce's former toxic diet, but we can learn a valuable lesson here. Bruce admitted to me that he was lucky and grateful that he didn't end up with diabetes, cancer, or any other major illness. The story of Bruce has a storybook ending (so far). In addition to totally cleaning out his system with his 7-Day "Alkalize & Energize" cleanse he did, the past 25 years Bruce has exercised on a regular basis and enjoys a healthy lifestyle where 80% of his diet is alkaline foods consisting mainly of vegetables, fruits, nuts, and sprouts. Bruce has another thing going for him in that his lovely wife is a strict vegetarian and an exercise buff (a 3rd degree black belt Taekwondo Do instructor) who works out 4 hours a day! We'll talk about this "support system" later, but it really helps to have someone in your household reinforcing your healthy lifestyle vs. an overweight roommate walking around the house smoking, drinking, and noshing on junk food all day. Another bonus besides having lots of energy and enjoying perfect health, Bruce and his wife each look at least 10 years younger than their real age!

"Physical 'age' is nonsense. It's much more important how old or young you decide to be in your own mind."
- unknown

CHAPTER SEVENTEEN (17):
The "Power" of Yoga!

Yoga is a physical, mental, and spiritual discipline, which originated in ancient India and can generate incredible power (stimulated from deep diaphramic breathing) as well as a powerful mind-body connection. Over the past 25 years, the number of yoga instructors and yoga centers has exploded in the U.S. and yoga has become popular as a physical system of health exercises. Long-term yoga practitioners for years have reported muscle–skeletal and mental health improvements. The benefits of yoga are almost too numerous to list, but here are a few Physiological Benefits: pulse & respiratory rate decreases, blood pressure decreases, cardiovascular & respiratory efficiency increases, gastrointestinal function normalizes, excretory functions improve, musculoskeletal flexibility and joint range of motion increase, lung capacity increases, overall muscle strength increases, posture and body alignment improves, energy level increases, weight normalizes (for most people a needed loss), sleep improves, pain decreases, balance improves (can sometimes improve vertigo). Psychological Benefits of yoga include but are not limited to: kinesthetic ("touch") awareness increases, mood improves, anxiety, stress, and depression decreases, concentration and memory improves, attention and attention deficit improves. Last but not least, Biochemical Benefits of yoga include: glucose & sodium decreases, LDL (the "bad" cholesterol) decreases, triglycerides decrease, hemoglobin increases, Lymphocyte (white blood cell) count increases, vitamin C increases, and serum protein increases.

If you've ever spoken with a registered or certified yoga instructor, in addition to being very energetic and health oriented people, they will often share some amazing stories. Here is one of them: DonnaLyn Giegerich MBA, CIC, RYT is a registered yoga instructor and a Kripalu yoga model in New Jersey where she teaches group classes as well as individual yoga instruction. DonnaLyn is also a global spokesperson, virtual columnist for a national health advocacy, mid life model and co-founder of Kick

Cancer Overboard (a nonprofit sending folks adversely affected by cancer on a free funfest cruise to Bermuda every year). She is also the President of DonnaLyn Giegerich Consulting, an empowerment speaking and training company providing customized coaching, keynotes, events and consulting for her corporate, professional and transitioning clients requesting leadership, mentoring & "skill up" solutions. This lady should be called "Superwoman" with all the superpowers she seems to possess! The interesting part of the story was several years ago and out of the blue, DonnaLyn found out she had the extremely rare Leiomyosarcoma malignant cancer (only 4 in 1 million people get this cancer)! It's an extremely resistant cancer and unfortunately not very responsive to chemotherapy or radiation. The best outcomes occur when the cancer can be removed surgically with wide margins early in the game. DonnaLyn had a large (baseball sized) tumor and had to have her entire kidney removed from her body during her first surgery. By sheer willpower and determination, DonnLyn ran, biked and swam through a year of surgical rehab, chemotherapy, and radiation when she then learned her husband Tom was diagnosed with a rare incurable cancer (talk about a double whammy)! Tom happens to be a close friend and fraternity brother of mine as well, and luckily he is a fighter who refused to give up on life. They both do yoga now on a regular basis for the incredible health benefits including the calming power and the deep breathing that leads to a plethora of health benefits including keeping cancer at bay! Undeterred by their circumstances, DonnaLyn and Tom have turned their challenges into a freeway of opportunity to serve others. Visit www.DonnaLyn.org if you want to learn more about her incredible story and the power of yoga that helped her maintain her now excellent health. Once again, don't take my word... ask any of your friends or neighbors who take yoga how they feel and hopefully one day in the near future, you can also feel the "power" or yoga. One yoga session or class might just change your life!

CHAPTER EIGHTEEN (18):
Understanding the Lymphatic System

Directly affected by deep diaphramic breathing is your body's critical lymphatic system of which is a brief overview here. As mentioned, the pulmonary system has a pump (the lungs), the circulatory system has its pump (the heart), but the lymphatic system (one of your body's most critical) has no pump. Here is Merriam-Webster's definition of lymph: "a usually clear coagulable fluid that passes from intercellular spaces of body tissue into the lymphatic vessels, is discharged into the blood by way of the thoracic duct and right lymphatic duct, and resembles blood plasma in containing white blood cells and especially lymphocytes". This lymph is basically the "waste" fluid and excess protein that has been squeezed out of the blood and drained from the tissue in microscopic blind-ended vessels called lymph capillaries to the thousands of lymph nodes. These lymph nodes filter the lymphatic fluid which contains white blood cells that attack and kill any infectious microorganisms and help remove toxins, poisons, etc. I highly recommend this YouTube video by BalancedHealthToday.com:
http://www.youtube.com/watch?v=XtkrN2hnK-o [18-1].
There are two (2) critically important messages to take away about your lymphatic system:

1) The more bad, acidic foods & drinks ("trash") you put into your body, the harder it is on your digestive system and also your lymphatic system.

2) The lymphatic system runs down a one-way street draining lymph from the tissue and returning it to the blood without a central pump. To facilitate the draining of this lymph, you can do exercise (activating muscle stimulation) and/or deep diaphramic breathing which stimulates your lymphatic system like a vacuum or pump.

These two points are reinforced by the fact that exercise makes you feel energized immediately and athletes on the average are 7 times less likely to get cancer! The lymphatic system is often compared to your city's sanitation service filtering out waste products, toxins, poisons and any material that could cause infections, disease or cancer. With modern day processed food and the massive quantities of meats, pastas, sodas, sugars, etc. we now consume, it's not a surprise that our lymphatic system (or sanitation system) is overtaxed. To make matters worse, most people in sedentary office jobs get distracted or don't make it a point of moving around every hour, so they often feel fatigued. If you start doing regular exercise on a daily basis (walking, running, cycling, hiking, lifting weights, tennis, etc.) you will feel more energized. Here is a great visual: instead of minimizing your trash by conservation, recycling, etc. and then putting this actual household trash into nice neat garbage bags at the end of your driveway so that the garbage men can easily pick it up every few days, you create an excess amount of trash and simply throw this trash all over your front yard. First of all your leaking trash with household toxins including today's cleaning products, bleaches, insecticides will start killing your front lawn, and secondly your garbage man is going to be overwhelmed! If enough trash starts piling up in your front yard and this goes on long enough, you will start having rats and other rodents come by until your front yard becomes a waste hazard. When people eat excess amounts of acidic, processed food and don't exercise (to stimulate their lymphatic system) this WILL lead to all kinds of disease, cancer, etc.

Finally another real danger of your lymphatic system not working properly (or you not helping your lymphatic system work properly) is edema, which is a swelling in part of your body (often your legs, arms, or even fingers) where excess lymph fluid is not disposed of properly. This is a serious problem and you should see a doctor immediately! This problem is often seen with older people who have a bad diet to begin with and if their health declines, they can often end up in a wheelchair which make there bodies even more immobile, which often leads them into a downward health spiral.

CHAPTER NINETEEN (19):
A Healthy Example (Mentor) in Your Life

The first time I learned how powerful "diet & exercise" were, I was shocked as this unfolded on national television. It all started innocently one day when I was walking through Universal Studios theme park in Orlando. A representative from America's Health Network spotted me and invited me to go on a television show called "Your Fitness Age". The premise of the show was to find out how "fit" people were in comparison to their real age. During the commercial breaks of the show, a health expert would give health tips to the contestants and the studio audience members. Never being one to shy away from any competition, I jumped at the chance to prove to the world how "fit" I was. I passed the initial questionnaire and then the network physicians & trainers ran a battery of tests on me including time exercises, flexibility measurements, lung capacity, blood pressure, a blood test, etc. The staff tallied up all my initial results and showed my results written on a clipboard to the show producer who shook his head in confusion. He ordered all the tests re-done one more time. I went through another 15 minutes of all these tests after which the producer shook his head once again and commented, "This is interesting... I have never seen this." Without any smiles on their faces, I assumed there might have been a problem like a pulmonary condition, cancer, etc. I begged someone to tell me something, but they were all tight-lipped stating they would reveal the results on the TV show next month if I wanted to come back and be a guest on the show. To make a long story short, a month later I waited in the green room for the longest half-hour of my life before stepping onto the set of "Your Fitness Age". I was nervous on one hand, but also confident that my daily exercise regimen along with regular juicing would prove me to be a healthy guest on the show. The host named Clark looked like an Olympic athlete and when he introduced me on the show, he boldly remarked: "We have NEVER seen these kind of results on the show before with anybody we have done all these tests." Making me sweat another minute or so, Clark finally revealed in almost all categories I had "the youngest fitness age of anyone they had on the show to date". **At the time I was 35 years old, but I had the fitness age of 17 (which was 16 years younger then my real age)!** I was not only relieved, but ecstatic that my daily exercise & balanced diet was working beyond my wildest dreams! I share this story not to brag, but to impress upon you that the five (5) major areas discussed in the book really DO work and can deliver amazing results.

My whole life, I've had a great role model (my oldest sister Niki) who showed me that a good diet & exercise plan really do work. Although almost 10 years older than me, Niki was often introduced to our friends as my "younger" sister. After coming back to the east coast from California (and later Mexico) where she lived for many years, she practiced mostly a vegetarian diet (eating organic, before it was the in-thing), and jogged, biked, or practiced yoga just about every single day. Even now (almost 60 years old) with a crazy work schedule of 50 – 60 hours a week, raising two daughters, and many more commitments I couldn't begin to list here, she never makes excuses about not having time to exercise. Even living in New Jersey in the winter (when it's dark in the morning and often 30 degrees outside before work), she will wake up an hour earlier so that she can get a 3 – 5 mile run in after she does her stretches and calisthenics. Her daily breakfast consists of a large fruit smoothie or 100% vegetable juice in contrast to the standard breakfast (coffee & danishes) that most of her co-workers choose. She literally looks like she could be 45 – 50 (10 – 15 years younger than her real age)! In addition, her energy level is through the roof... I don't think I've met anyone more energetic in my life. Now if you don't have an energetic sister like I do to serve as a role model, perhaps you have an aunt, uncle, or a cousin who can serve as an example of great health. If nobody in your extended family has consistent healthy habits, hire a personal trainer who not only talks a good game, but who also "walks the talk". My recommendation is to hire a trainer who looks like an Olympic athlete and has earned the "results" you yourself want. If you don't have the money for a personal trainer, the best starting point would be to go to your public library and get a few fitness books from authors who are true athletes. Learn from someone else who has gotten lasting results you are looking for. Once again CONGRATULATIONS for investing your time and money into reading this book as you are among the 1% of people who are taking action towards perfect health, and not part of the 99% who keep the same habits that got you overweight, sick, or fatigued. Good luck in finding an inspiring example (someone with excellent health & energy) in your life and gaining back your own perfect health!

⇔ SUBSTITUTE: If you need an energy boost, don't think about any beverage or food, or even anything with calories. Substitute instead 2 – 3 minutes of deep diaphramic breathing. By flooding your entire body with oxygen, you will instantly feel better and you can do this while standing (best), sitting, or even while driving in your car.

SECTION III:
HYDRATE

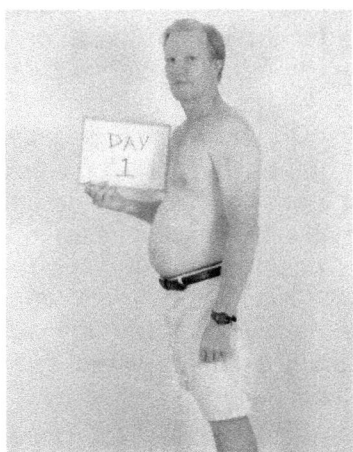

Author Scott duPont starting an "Alkalize & Energize" cleanse.
Notice how tight the shorts & belt are in this photo.

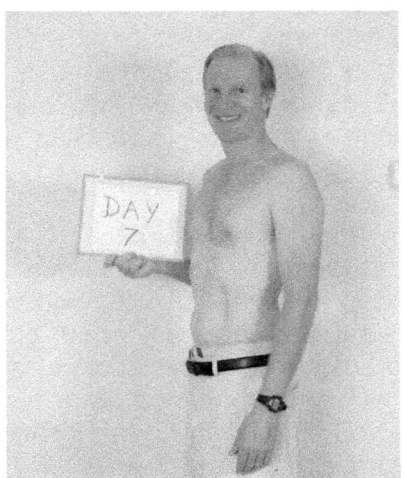

On day 7, I was totally "Energized!"
I lost 2" in the waist after the cleanse.

CHAPTER TWENTY (20):
<u>Observe Those Who Don't Drink Water</u>

Before moving on to the heart of this section of "Hydration", picture two images in your mind... one a dry, parched Arizona desert and another image a lush, rainy part of the country such as Seattle, Washington (where it rains over 150 days a year). Do you want your body to be dry, brittle, & shriveled up or healthy, vital and strong? Now if this analogy doesn't work for you, visualize an older alcoholic or wino (anyone who drinks at least 5 – 6 drinks every single day). This could be a drunken bum on the street, or perhaps a family member who is an alcoholic. If this person smokes, it will intensify the result as smokers usually do not drink as much water as non-smokers and smoke accelerates the drying effect of cells in your body. Compare the "alcoholic" to any healthy person you know who drinks lots of water. Take a good look at the wrinkled and shriveled skin of the alcohol drinker-smoker vs. the person who drinks lots of water every day combined with lots of water-rich vegetables & fruits. If you take a few minutes to do this observation (even someone as young as in their 40s or 50s), the need to drink water will be crystal clear! Since your body is approximately 70% water, it needs an abundance of water for your cells, tissues, organs and your entire body to function properly and be healthy.

You might have heard your mother (or another family member) when you were young tell you to drink lots of water to hydrate your body, so this should NOT be a new concept. However, it is very easy in our busy lives to start drinking "flavored" water, sodas, coffee, and other acidic liquids which will counter-act any water you are drinking, so make sure you start applying this concept of hydrating with pure water every single day!

CHAPTER TWENTY-ONE (21):
WATER... the River of ALL Life!

Our planet, our bodies, and our cells, etc. are composed mostly of water. As mentioned, approximately 70% of our body is water! Our brains are composed of 85% water and even our bones contain 10 – 15% water. Water is the perfect conductor of electricity, especially when our bodies are "alkalized" as discussed earlier in the book. Water is also the perfect solvent. Water makes up a huge content of our blood, which is why blood is often called the "river of life". Plasma is often 95% water, so you can imagine how critical water is to a healthy body as your heart pumps approximately 2,000 gallons of blood each day through your body! A normal baby has an 80% water content, while an old person drinking lots of soda, coffee, alcohol, etc. might be closer to 60% water content. The reason why morticians embalm dead bodies is by the time older people die (and afterwards), they have much less water content. The morticians will pump water and other chemicals into the body to make it more presentable for a viewing and to temporarily preserve the body of a deceased person. Since your body is made up of so much water, it is only common sense that you should drink lots of water every day. Liquids such as coffee, soft drinks, fruit flavored drinks, sport drinks, and cocktails do NOT hydrate or cleanse your body, and in fact they have the opposite effect. In addition to drinking plenty of pure water (NOT these new "flavored" water drinks), it's common sense to eat lots of "water-rich" foods. What exactly are water-rich foods? Keep reading and you'll find out in the next chapter.

CHAPTER TWENTY-TWO (22):
High Water Content (Water-Rich) Foods

If you look at the "SAD" (Standard American Diet), of which most people in the country partake, about 80% consists of processed or enriched foods, meats, dairy, wheat, pasta, etc., none of which are water-rich. Once again, the beverages consumed by the majority of the population (influenced by mass advertising and what is most readily available) are NOT helping hydrate your body. It should be no surprise when these above listed foods are accompanied by soda, coffee, milk, etc. they are contributing to the current health epidemic. As optimistic as I am about a lot of things, I truly fear that the health epidemic in this country will get worse the next few years before its gets better based mainly based upon the younger people I saw come up to my Medco table the past few years already taking several different prescription drugs.

A powerful exercise I encourage you to do is to write down a list (an inventory) of all the food you ate the previous day and BE HONEST. My guess is that unless you are fully cognizant and focused on eating water-rich foods, less than 50% of your diet is from water-rich foods. Is this you? Not only does this diet fatigue your body (and a major reason why many people feel tired all the time), but this diet is a recipe for allergies, illness, and eventually cancer. If you find that less than 25% of your diet consists of water-rich foods, this is suicide! Make sure you close this book right now and do an inventory of what you ate and drank the last 24 hours. By looking at a list of everything that passed between your lips the past day, this will be an eye-opening experience and just being aware of your percentage of water-rich foods should inspire you to switch over to healthier, water-rich foods which your water-rich body is craving. This is why people are often thirsty. But make no mistake, your body is not thirsty for soda, coffee, or milk. Your body is thirsty for water!

So what are water-rich foods? Almost all vegetables and fruits. The juicier a fruit or vegetable is (when you cut into them), the better. For example: when you cut into watermelons, oranges, peaches, cucumbers, beets, tomatoes, you can see the water dripping out. These are very water-rich foods as are almost all fruits & vegetables. Sprouts & many seeds are also water-rich foods.

Dried fruits like raisins and cranberries are NOT water-rich, so even though these are healthy foods, they should be eaten in moderation. Many dried fruits are also high in sugar content, and while a small amount of natural sugar is OK, be very careful to limit the quantities. Eating a salad at every meal is the easiest way to start boosting your ratio of water in your daily diet. Remember that almost all these vegetables, fruits, sprouts, etc. are also alkaline which is a good step towards a healthy and energetic body. Once you change your diet by hydrating with lots of water and ensuring the majority of your diet consists of water-rich foods, your cells, your organs, and your entire body will function much more efficiently. Since water is a great conductor of electricity, you will feel more energy after a few glasses of pure lemon water than if you haven't had any water all day. Most importantly your blood (the "river of life") will be much more efficient and will be able to carry more oxygen to all parts of your body including your brain making you feel more energetic and alert. Once you understand this concept of hydrating your body and how it makes every part of your body operate more efficiently, it makes perfect sense!

"It's bizarre that the produce manager is more important to my children's health than the pediatrician."
- **Meryl Streep**

CHAPTER TWENTY-THREE (23):
What Water Should You Drink? Alkaline!

This chapter has been condensed and simplified. If you would like more detailed information on water, there are books on the subject of the best drinking water and of course you can do your own research on the internet. Since the last chapter just discussed "water-rich" foods, a portion of the water your body needs should come from those vegetables, fruits, sprouts, etc. As far as actual drinking water, if money is no object, you can buy alkaline water from a health food store or buy an alkaline filtration system for your home. These systems can run over $1,000 and since this book is NOT sponsored by any manufacturers; we're not endorsing one system over another, but Kangen and Lifeionizers are companies worth researching. If you have the money for a complete system, do your homework and ask other people who have been using their system for an extended period of time. Never be afraid to ask for references. An important note here: just because you might be buying and drinking alkaline water (or making it yourself at home with a filtration system and alkalizing with lemons – see below), this alone is NOT a magical cure. Alkaline water is a very important piece of the overall health puzzle, but if 80% or more of your diet (your other beverages and foods) is not alkaline, you will NOT get (or stay) healthy from drinking alkaline water alone.

If you live in certain parts of the country (New York City for example), the tap water can be exceptional. Your local water utility can provide you with detailed information about your water quality as a consumer. If your residence has a deep well, that is also an excellent water source. In most cases you might want to buy an inexpensive pitcher filtration (Brita and ZERO water seem to be the most popular brands). Once again shop around for the best product you can find. These pitcher filtration systems can be found on-line as well as the big discount stores like Target & Wal-Mart and run well under $50 including the actual filters to get you started. Once you have your water ready to pour into your clean glass, you should add 2 or 3 lemon slices, which will have an alkalizing effect on your water. I also add one ice cube to every glass of water. A single ice cube will not chill your water very much, but as the solid-state is changed to a liquid-state, this will add some energy to your water. While writing this chapter, I am on my 3rd glass of lemon water early this morning and have an abundance of energy. Why not start every morning by alkalizing and energizing your system this way?

A very important note is NOT to fall for the marketing trap of all these new bottled water beverages which are marketed as "water", but often contain a wide variety of additional ingredients, ranging from natural or artificial flavors, sugars, sweeteners, caffeine, vitamins, minerals and other additives or enhancements. Just stick to regular water (as described above), which costs very little, but will add big benefits to your health!

"The longer I live the less confidence I have in drugs & the greater is my confidence in the regulation and administration of diet and regimen."
- John Redman Coxe, 1800

CHAPTER TWENTY-FOUR (24):
More and More Vegetarians

Being an actor by trade, I'm always observing people very carefully. I look at people's outer appearance and skin (since that is what the camera sees) and over the past few years I have this uncanny ability to guess who is a vegetarian (most of the time). One day I was working on a TV game show "The Pyramid" that my friend Mike Richards is producing and hosting, and I was sitting in the audience next to a beautiful girl named Dianne who was not only pretty, but very lean with flawless skin. I figured she was in her mid 30s. Dianne was telling me stories about her world travels, her different careers, and then she started going on and on about her tours in Vietnam as a nurse. This girl (actually a middle aged lady) had done two tours in Vietnam! She was actually 25+ years older than she looked! The only thing Dianne told me that did NOT shock me was that she had become a vegetarian 30 years ago.

While I'm not 100% vegetarian (or a vegan), I applaud the growing number of vegetarians for several reasons, primarily because eating fresh vegetables, fruits, sprouts, nuts, etc. is a very healthy lifestyle. Every vegetarian I've met (including Dianne) looks healthy, appears energetic, and usually has glowing, radiant skin. In addition to hydrating by drinking water, vegetarians are getting a large quantity of water (in essence hydrating) through all the water-rich vegetables, fruits, and sprouts they eat. I've shifted my diet the past few years to 90% vegetarian and in addition to "alkalizing" my body with these alkaline natural vegetarian foods, I'm also "hydrating" my cells every time I eat water-rich veggies & fruits. If you don't have any close family members or friends who are vegetarians, or if you think that vegetarians are unhealthy or simply crazy, don't be too quick to judge. Some of the most energetic & healthy people I've ever met or worked with are vegetarians or vegans. To list a few famous people you probably know or have seen on television, they include: Ryan Seacrest, Paul McCartney, Alexandra Paul, Elizabeth Berkley, Christian Bale, Tobey Maguire, James

Cameron, Tony Robbins, Bill Walton, Bill Clinton, and Brad Pitt. You would be surprised at the list of professional athletes who are vegetarians as well including: Heisman trophy winner Ricky Williams, Atlanta Falcons tight end Tony Gonzalez, legendary tennis champion Chris Everett, UFC champion Mac Danzig, and NY Jets icon Joe Namath. Dr. William Casteli of the Framingham Heart Study reported in his study that "vegetarians have the lowest cholesterol counts, and the lowest rates of cancer and heart disease. Those with the lowest cholesterol levels also outlived everyone else." [24-1]

The main concern uneducated people have about going vegetarian, is that they think they can't get enough nutrition or protein. I strongly suggest you research how much protein you can get from different all-natural sources including spinach, mushrooms, sprouts, seeds, and of course nuts. There is no way in this short book I can get into all the details, but there are books out there as well as information on-line where you can get more info, including great menus if this is a lifestyle you choose. As mentioned, I've never felt better since 90% of my diet is alkaline consisting of a primarily water-rich vegetarian diet. I occasionally eat meat when offered to me on special social occasions including the Holidays, but I almost never buy or prepare any meat dishes myself.

The other reason to consider being a vegetarian (besides being great for your health) is for the health of our planet. With the rapidly growing population and limited resources, climate change, etc. we're all going to face more food and water shortages if we continue the course we're on. There are several great documentaries out including "Last Call at the Oasis" and "Tapped" which explore how severe this water problem is becoming. I would also suggest reading one or both of John Robbins' best selling books: May All Be Fed and The Food Revolution. In these books, the passionate author (who was constantly sick as a child eating lots of his family's Baskin-Robbins ice cream as well as meat, cheese, etc.), not only talks about how he found true health, but John shares compelling information about how inefficient (and what a great waste of resources) it is for us to eat a meat favored diet vs. a plant based diet.

Consider this mind-blowing statistic straight from the Water Education Foundation. **It takes 2,464 gallons of water to produce 1 pound of California beef, while it only takes 23 gallons of water to produce 1 pound of lettuce!** [24-2]. This is an INSANE and UNSUSTAINABLE way to feed the world especially with millions of new meat lovers around the world (including the booming populations of China and other Asian countries) switching from a vegetable & rice based diet to a fast food diet. As you may have read, there are thousands of new McDonald's & Burger King restaurants being added every year overseas. By the way, the health of the Chinese population (while not nearly as bad as here in America) is declining fast including millions of new cases of Type II diabetes being reported in China alone each year!

The final reason to consider going vegetarian (or vegan) is that **vegetarians live an average of six to ten years longer than the rest of the population!** [24-3] If you're still not sold on eating more veggies, please read and ponder this quote from one of the smartest men in the history of the world. Albert Einstein had the foresight many years to ago to write: "Nothing will benefit human health and increase the chances for survival of life on earth as much as the evolution of a vegetarian diet". Now that was one smart man!

⇔ SUBSTITUTE: The next time you're thirsty, stop and think about what your body really needs…water! Don't just grab a bottled beverage. Substitute a nice tall glass of water with a twist of lemon (described in Chapter 7). You'll give you body what it really needs while quenching your thirst.

SECTION IV:
EXERCISE

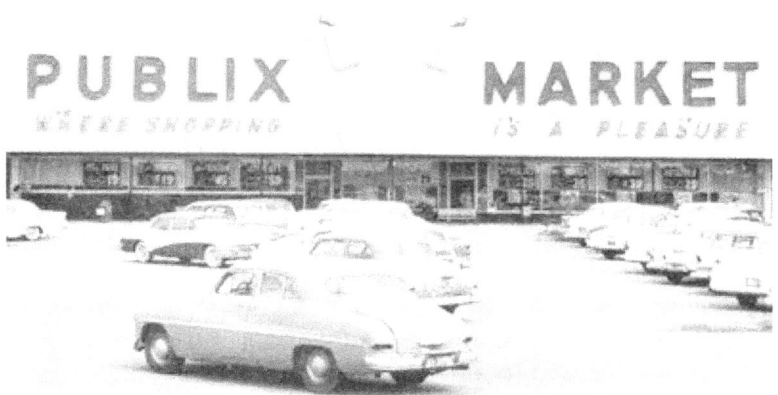

Just a few decades ago, Publix (a great super market)
was actually called a Super "Market".

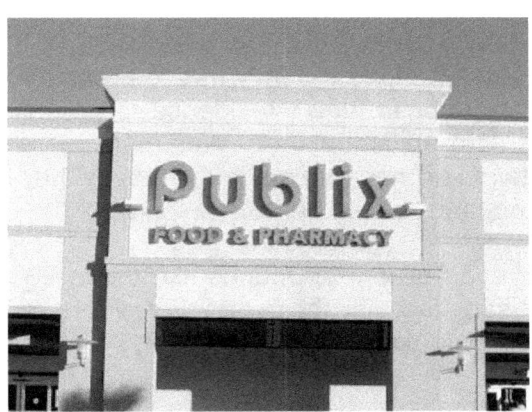

The new slogan for Publix: "Food & Pharmacy". A sign of the
times of many grocery stores, since an increasing portion of their
business is from their pharmacy.

CHAPTER TWENTY-FIVE (25):
<u>Childhood Obesity...an Epidemic!</u>

In just the past 20 years, we've created an epidemic in this country where 13 million children and teenagers are now obese, and that number is growing fast! [25-1] People often talk about this epidemic like it was created by some outside force. The cold, hard fact is that MOST obese kids bring obesity on themselves (and in many cases the ignorance or neglect from their parents). What I mean by that is that MOST kids are simply consuming many more calories (and sugar) than they are burning off every day. Just look at the increased portion sizes of today's food along with the reduction of sports programs, outdoor activities, and other exercise. While you probably read the statistics and stories in the news headlines every day, let me share just two recent horrific ones:

1) An Ohio third-grader weighing more than 200 pounds was taken from his family and placed into foster care after county social workers said his mother wasn't doing enough to control his weight. The Cleveland 8 year old was considered severely obese and at risk for many diseases including diabetes and hypertension. [25-2]

2) Emergency workers recently had to break through a wall of a morbidly obese teen's residence to get her out of her room and into an ambulance. Workmen busted a hole in the upstairs of her house to remove the 835-pound teenage girl and rushed her to a hospital. [25-3]

I couldn't even dream up stories like these 20 years ago! Yet the sad fact is these tragic events are actually happening to our kids today.

Even being moderately obese (kids who are just 15 – 20 lbs. overweight) is a tragedy that often creates a downward spiral. For those of you who have ever been to a gym, can you imagine harnessing a 20lb. dumbbell on your little kid to carry around every single day? Once these kids pack on a little extra weight, they are less likely to exercise, run, or participate in sports. They are more likely to find comfort on the sofa where they can play video games all day long while sipping on unlimited sodas and ice cream that many parents allow them to consume. Then when the caffeine and sugar wears off, the kids will grab one of these new energy drinks loaded with even more caffeine mixed with taurine, ephedrine, carnitine, phosphoric acid, guarana, citric acid, ascorbic acid, and tons of sugar. Once pumped up again, the kids will waddle over from the couch to their computer where they will e-mail, IM, or connect with friends on the many social media sites for hours on end. While very sad, it is only common sense that all these kids (millions of them) are now getting obese, while developing type II diabetes, high blood pressure, allergies, and many other ailments. If you are a parent reading this book, take a long hard look at your kid and his or her health. In chapters 8 and 9, you can start turning your kids health around in just 7 days and help them progress to a healthier lifestyle. One of the best gifts I get is when someone calls or writes to tell me how they turned their child's health around in those 7 days of the "Alkalize & Energize" cleanse. If you have a child or teenager with any health issues that this book changes, please let me know. I would love to hear your success story!

"There's lots of people in this world who spend so much time watching their health that they haven't the time to enjoy it."
- Josh Billings

CHAPTER TWENTY-SIX (26):
Observe Those Who Move!

Tony Robbins has a profound saying that: "Motion Creates Emotion!" It's a fact that once you get your body in motion, you create momentum and speed up your body's metabolism. This motion creates energy, which can last for hours on end and often carry you through the whole day. On the other hand, once you sit your butt down in your chair (hopefully not your Lazy-Boy TV lounger), it tends to stick there. Later in life when your body stops moving completely, you are DEAD! Along these thoughts, I feel compelled to share a tragic story, which happened right in my own neighborhood. Whenever I don't have an early call time for a film shoot, I head out my door between 6 - 7:00am for a powerwalk (where I do deep breathing for about 10 minutes), build up to a nice easy jog for 10 minutes, and then wrap up the last 5 minutes or so in a fast paced run where I shout out my daily incantations. Talk about an incredible way to start the day, you should try it... you will feel incredible! Anyway, here's where the sad story comes in. In my neighborhood, I noticed a really obese, bald guy, who looked like he may have been in his 50s. I would see this gentleman 2 – 3 times a week either coming or going to Jon's grocery store, which is only two blocks away. Literally it is a 2- minute walk from his house directly to Jon's. It is actually further and takes longer with the stop signs and traffic lights to drive to the grocery store vs. walking. Now I never want to judge people who have major disabilities or handicaps, but this man although very obese (probably 5'10" and 240 lbs.), and bow-legged, he could easily walk to his van. His daily routine (even on Sundays) was to waddle out of his front door of his house about 30 steps over to his van, climb up into the cab and drive across the street where he bought the daily newspaper and a large cup of coffee. Over the past 3 years I observed very carefully the downfall of this man. After about a year, the 30 foot walk (or shuffle) to his van was getting painfully slow and every few weeks it seemed to be more of a chore for him to actually climb into the driver's seat of the van. As strange as it seems, I also noticed that over time, he had aged and looked several years older. I was literally watching the slow, steady decline of this poor soul. This routine went on for about 2 years and then one day I noticed an old lady walk out to the van and she drove across the street to get his paper and coffee. I would see her from time to time the next few months perform this daily ritual of getting her husband's paper and coffee. A few months later, they sold the van and just recently I asked their neighbors what happened to this gentleman? It turns out he died! As tragic a story as this is, I literally watched this old man die over the course of the last 3 years. The moral of the story is exercise and just KEEP MOVING if you want to live!

Here's a different and truly inspiring story you've probably heard about involving a famous person who kept moving in order to live! Senator John McCain was shot down in Vietnam on October 26,1967 and fractured both arms and a leg ejecting from his aircraft. McCain suffered other injuries through repeated torture and beatings by his captives. He was eventually transported to the famous "Hanoi Hilton" prison where he spent almost 6 years including long stints in solitary confinement. Here's the relevant part of the story if you haven't read his incredible autobiography. No matter how bad the pain, dysentery, or how low his energy was, he made a conscious decision that he would exercise every single day. Even when he only had enough room to do push ups and sit-ups, or when he had a limited amount of energy to move his legs back and forth while swinging his arms, McCain would force his body to move every single day. McCain equated exercising every day as the only way to ensure that he would LIVE. Luckily his daily exercise regimen and his fortitude helped him survive until he was released on March 14, 1973. In his memoirs, he mentioned that every other fellow P.O.W. and prisoner he encountered at the Hanoi Hilton who did NOT EXERCISE (to keep moving their bodies) DIED!

You've probably heard the importance of exercise from your elementary school gym teacher, First Lady Michelle Obama (when she started her "Get Moving" campaign), or perhaps heard your doctor tell you to exercise. Yet MOST people do very little exercise including walking. The plethora of plasma television screens, computers, laptops, i-pods, smart phones, and video games might make us move our fingers, but not the rest of our bodies, hence the U.S. population is getting fatter and sicker every single year.

The next time you're in an office building, observe the 1% who will take the stairs up 5 flights of an office building vs. the 99% who crowd into office elevator with everyone else. If you're in an airport, observe the 10% of people who continue to walk on the moving sidewalks (or sometimes bypass the moving sidewalks all together) vs. the 90% majority who stand still. For those of you who love to go to the shopping mall, look at the 10% of people who walk rapidly up the stairs vs. the 90% who take the escalator or the elevator up to the 2nd level food court. Do you notice that many of the people who walk or climb the stairs are slimmer? Do these people seem to have more energy than the people stopped in their tracks clinging on to the escalator handrail? If you are one of those people who claim you "never have enough time to exercise", why not start tomorrow taking the stairs, or walking to the neighbor's house instead of driving the next time you have an errand. A little bit of daily exercise doesn't have to take a lot of time, but can go a long way to improving your health & energy levels. Keep reading because in chapter 31 we'll explore the concept of exercising using NET ("No Extra Time") time to move your body every day and become part of the 10% who move vs. the 90% who snooze!

"The doctor has been taught to be interested
not in health, but in disease.
What the public is taught is that health
is the cure for disease."
- Ashley Montagu

CHAPTER TWENTY-SEVEN (27):
How Did We Get So Out of Shape?

My brother Peter and I took my 13-year-old niece Sarah to Universal Studios theme park last summer. Sarah lives in Thailand and it was her first time to Orlando, Florida as well as her first time to a major theme park, which she really enjoyed. Before we entered the park, I pulled her aside and said: "Sarah, don't be alarmed, but notice how many really fat people you are going to see here today." A rough estimate we came up with is that at least 3 – 4 out of every 10 people were obese. She was shocked (as was I). In between waiting for our group to get on and off the rides, I decided to count the number of little electric scooters that the park rented out to really obese people (not just to old or handicapped people like they used to). In just 20 minutes, I counted thirty-five (35) grossly obese people driving around on these scooters and almost all of them were well over 250 – 300 lbs! Once again, I never want to belittle people who lost their legs, or have some sort of genetic disease, or handicap keeping them from walking, but it was clear that day that many of those 35 people were simply grossly overweight which prevented them from walking properly. That was a real eye opener! Time magazine now reports that there is not a single state in the union with an obesity rate of less than 20%, and the CDC found many states have obesity rates of well over 30%! [27-1]

So how did we get so out of shape as a country and as a society? The main reason is most Americans simply do NOT exercise! In fact, only about 5% of American adults do some type of vigorous physical activity on any given day, according to the results of a new Health Day study. [27-2] If you look at the history of mankind, ever since the caveman days, people were always moving and quite active in terms of "hunting and gathering" their own food. Fast forward thousands of years to the modern era in the 1800s and the 1st half of the 1900s, there was still a lot of manual labor, including farmers who worked their land, and far fewer cars and other modern transportation devices. Even in the 1960s and 1970s when I grew up as a kid, a significant amount of the population still worked in factories and did manual labor & service jobs. It was also common for most kids to walk or ride bicycles to school. My bike ride was almost 6 miles to school (12 miles round trip) which I did most days unless it was too cold, raining, or snowing. Once I got to school, there was mandatory gym class & all kinds of sports (that all kids HAD to participate in), and at least two different recess periods where we would rush outside to the playground to ride swings, play four square, dodge ball, etc. Then after an exhausting football or basketball practice, I would ride my bike back home 6 miles to play outside for another hour or so before dinner. If my brother & I got our homework done (and checked by our parents), we were only then allowed to play a game of basketball where my stepfather had set up a backboard & outdoor lights for us. All the current day conveniences like TV remote controls, cordless phones, and electric windows in cars were not that common 30 – 40 years ago. People watching TV would have to jump up from their chair to answer the phone or change the channel. People used to manual shift gears in their cars, wrestle with manual steering columns (before power assisted steering), and physically crank open the windows in their cars. If you look around your house, there are now hundreds of modern day conveniences like electric can openers, microwave ovens, etc. that make life easier but reduce or eliminate many of the physical activities we used to do. It's clear that there are fewer farmers, fewer manufacturing jobs, fewer manual labor service jobs in our society and more and more people working in cubicles or people telecommuting from their homes with their but planted in a chair for 8 hours staring at a computer screen. For kids, many physical education and gym classes do not exist anymore due to budget cuts. I've witnessed first hand kids coming home from school to either text their friends on their smart phones or plop on the couch for hours at a time playing video games or watching YouTube. I applaud what Michele Obama is doing to try to fight this obesity epidemic (especially with kids and teens). With her fitness initiative, her team has created a great website (www.LetsMove.org) for kids and their parents to get moving towards a healthier lifestyle!

In addition to this major shift (especially the last 40 years) reducing physical activity for people, the other component which has gotten the general population so out of shape is the amount of processed, refined, acidic foods that we eat as a modern society as mentioned earlier in section I. I am horrified whenever I visit a public school and see Pizza Hut and Taco Bell as lunch options, knowing how little of those calories most kids will burn off with exercise. Tony Robbins (who is doing great work to educate people of all ages about nutrition and reclaiming vibrant health & energy) shared a recent report that "many of today's children are eating 30 times mores sugar than their grandparents did"! The other component of poor food is the size portions that have slowly grown over the years. When I was a young kid, once a month I got a special treat of a Coca-Cola. For anyone old enough to remember the Coca-Cola bottles were only 8oz. and have become quite a collector's item today since they are such a rarity. The old portion sizes are a contrast to the 32 oz. and 64 oz. soda sizes, which are so common today. In chapter 11, you saw the detailed table comparing the massive increase in portion sizes for different kinds of food and drinks. I think you get the picture, but to summarize, as a society we are not exercising (or even moving our bodies) like we used to, and we are eating and drinking much larger portions of poor nutritional quality food. Fewer calories burned and more calories consumed is a recipe for disaster!

"Sickness is the vengeance of nature
for the violation of her laws."
- **Charles Simmons**

CHAPTER TWENTY-EIGHT (28):
A Healthy Body Assessment

Now is the time to be completely HONEST with yourself. Don't use softeners or listen to your family or close friends who tell you that you're in "pretty good shape", or that you're "not really overweight, but just big-boned". Remember in terms of your body and your health, what is "common" now, is not necessarily "normal". If you took the time to read this book and got this far, congratulations! You obviously want to improve your health, or perhaps want to reclaim the energy you enjoyed as a young kid. For an assessment of how healthy your lifestyle and your body is, here are ten (10) simple questions to ask yourself:

1) Are you your ideal body weight?
(Calculate your BMI "Body Mass Index" and make sure you are well under 25 BMI).

2) Are you taking multiple prescription (or over the counter) drugs on a daily basis?

3) Do you ever get winded when walking long distances or climbing a flight of stairs?

4) Has your blood pressure elevated over time?

5) Do you ever have indigestion or acid reflux?

6) Do you occasionally have constipation or diarrhea?

7) Do you often feel fatigued at work, or at the end of the day?

8) Do you have allergies, sinus problems, or a persistent cough?

9) Do you have MAJOR cravings (chocolate, sweets, alcohol, or coffee)?

10) Do you have any cuts, scrapes, or scabs that don't completely heal up in a few days?

If you answered YES to 3 or more of these questions, be HONEST with yourself and keep reading the rest of this book. Taking more prescriptions (or over the counter drugs) is not the answer. I also recommend you go back and re-read chapter 6 about the effects of acid on your health which contributes to most of today's health problems. A great deal of these symptoms (warning signs) can be completely eliminated when you "alkalize & energize" your body. A few people we showed these questions to did not answer them all because they did not know their blood pressure numbers or their BMI index. Here's a quick tip: many supermarkets and drug stores (that want to sell blood pressure medication and other profitable prescription drugs) have a blood pressure machine where you check your blood pressure for free. There are now free BMI calculators on the internet (just do a Google search) and plug in your height & weight.

As my good friend and author Monroe Mann says "no excuses!" Take the time to do this quick assessment before you move on to the next chapter to find out what the new view on health care will hopefully look like.

"Most of the limits we put on our bodies
start in our minds."
- unknown

CHAPTER TWENTY-NINE (29):
<u>Finally, A New View on Health Care!</u>

No matter how bleak things look for the future, there is hope as there is a new view on health care by many health professionals, companies who contribute to the cost of their employees health care, and by human resource administrators. It's called "Consumer Driven Health Care" (CDHC) and it's a new shift for individual employees (consumers of health care services) to take responsibility for THEIR own health! This past year I've seen some companies present a health insurance option where employees can significantly lower their monthly premiums by agreeing to pay the first $2,500.00 out of their pocket. This is a new and radical concept, which saves employees and contributing companies money each month, but most importantly it changes the way employees (the consumers) view and use their health insurance. Here's an example: if an employee has a comprehensive health care plan with a $5 co-pay on their prescriptions, and a $10 co-pay to visit their doctor, and free emergency room visits, there's not much of a financial deterrent for the employee to not use the plan like crazy. Now if that same employee has a plan option with a $25 co-pay on prescriptions and has to pay 100% of the cost of each doctor office visit and an initial $100 emergency room fee as well as all costs (capped at $2,500.00 per year), there is a HUGE incentive for this employee to really focus on his her health and perhaps think about a better diet, more exercise and any preventive steps so in the long run they don't have as many medical expenses. The $2,500.00 cap is insurance to protect employees from a catastrophic illness and most of these plans will allow employees free office visits to test for any "preventative" health measures. For example: prostrate screenings, mammograms and colonoscopies for employees after a certain age are still free to encourage employees to routinely check for cancer, etc. to catch any serious health issues early.

Some forward thinking companies embracing CHDC (like Fidelity Investments) are now also offering discounts (or in some cases) FREE gym memberships & wellness classes as incentives to get their employees in better shape. One company I consulted with even gave away a $250.00 pre-paid VISA card in addition to a free gym membership if the employee did a simple 30-minute health assessment! I saw another company offer a contest including a paid vacation with a free cruise (valued at $5,000.00) for a team of two people who lost the most weight! At the end of the year, both team members would be rewarded with a paid 7-day vacation with their spouses (or significant others)! This company in the 1st week had 30 teams sign up to take the weight loss challenge which fostered team work, a major commitment to personal health, boosted morale for all company employees, while gaining great PR both inside and outside the company showing a caring company dedicated to the health and welfare of their employees! Hopefully more consumers and companies will think long term about getting healthier (which will reduce health care costs), as we are headed for a financial cliff very soon. Just least decade, the U.S. spent a few hundred million dollars annually on health care, while last year, heath care costs in the U.S. soared to $2.6 trillion! [29-1] That is NOT a typo and the sicker America gets, the higher these health care costs will keep climbing!

If the U.S. doesn't embrace CDHC (or some sort a new view on health care), our country might well default on its debt in the next ten (10) years. If you think I'm exaggerating or being melodramatic, ask any government official or any human resources person you know, and they'll tell you about the staggering cost (and exponential cost increases) of health care in just the last few years. Health care costs are not just growing by 2 - 3% each year, or by the cost of annual inflation, but these costs are now growing by over 5 % most years during the past decade and will continue to increase even more as our population gets fatter, more toxic, and sicker. Kaiser Family Foundation, a nonprofit research group that tracks employer-sponsored health insurance on a yearly basis, shows that the average annual premium for family coverage through an employer reached $15,073 in 2011, an increase of 9 percent over the previous year! [29-2]

As mentioned, being on the front lines (working for Medco) I've spoken to over 12,000 people who visited the Medco table at health fairs asking me questions about their prescription drugs. The majority of people I answered questions for were taking maintenance medications (such as blood pressure, cholesterol, anti-acid medications, etc.) and switched over, or will be switching over to mail order where they can expand their prescription supply to 90 days vs. a 30 day supply which the retail pharmacy normally dispenses. Here's a frightening observation: just 7 or 8 years ago, I would normally consult with older people (in their 50s or 60s) or even older retirees taking multiple prescriptions. It was absolutely shocking to see more and more young people in their late 20s and 30s now taking these "maintenance" medications. It breaks my heart to see these young people already taking multiple prescriptions for different ailments on a daily basis. One day last year, over a dozen people came up to me who have cancer or who have an immediate family member with cancer. This rapid increase of sick, diseased people just breaks my heart.

I don't usually generalize, but the health of the majority of Medco patients 8 years ago was significantly better the health of most people I spoke to yesterday (August 21, 2012) at the Medco table. I have a clear picture of much thinner, healthier vibrant folks with smiles on their faces who would come by the Medco table stating: "I don't take any prescriptions yet!" I now notice more obese people (many who seem fatigued), and of course many more now taking multiple prescriptions. Being on the front lines like this is what caused me to study and research the current state of our health care and finally write this book. If you're lucky enough to have a job which offers any kind of insurance, and if a CDHC program makes sense for you, please look into this option and start taking more responsibility for YOUR health!

CHAPTER THIRTY (30): "PLAN" Your Exercise!

Smart people plan their careers and futures starting with what schools (and classes) they're going to attend. Most families plan their vacations. People with great relationships (at least lasting ones), plan and work on their relationships for years. Rich people (who don't win the lottery) plan their business goals along with their long-term investment strategies to obtain the level of wealth they want to achieve. Olympic athletes set their targets & regimented training schedules for years before they qualify for the Olympics and then rehearse in their minds their final routines thousands of times in addition to the physical practice they do. Why should it be any different for you if you want to achieve excellent health? The fact is, it's no different than any other area of your life. If you want to achieve weight loss, gain more defined muscles, have longer endurance, or increased vitality & energy, then you'll need a plan. This book does NOT outline a specific plan for you as everyone is different and there literally are hundreds of different types of exercises and plans out there. However, this book does offer dozens of specific tips and strategies that you can start implementing to achieve your health & fitness goals including the 7-Day "Alkalize & Energize" program in chapter 9. For those folks more ambitious who choose a long term work out program, and you've never done any regular exercise or fitness routines before (3rd grade gym class does not count), you might look into joining a gym or a fitness club. Perhaps look into your local community center to see if there are any exercise classes you could join on a regular basis? Maybe you want to get a trainer or hire a coach to help reinforce you and guide you towards improved fitness?

Whatever plan you decide upon and map out for your plan, here are **Three (3) Tips for Success**:

1) **Write out your plan** on paper (or on your computer). Don't just keep the plan up in your head. It can be a simple 1 – 2 page written plan you come up with, but write your plan down including what action steps you're going to commit to in

terms of exercise, even if you start off by just walking!

2) **Find the underlying reason WHY you will commit to your plan** whether it's walking 5 times a week, going to the gym twice a week, bicycling to work once a week instead of driving every day. If your underlying reason is to so that you stay healthy enough to see all your grandchildren graduate from college or get married, those are powerful emotional reasons to get healthy.

3) **Share your plan with your family, a good friend, or even a co-worker**. As soon as you tell someone else your plan and what you are doing, you now have "leverage" in that from time to time that family member or friend will ask how your plan is going. A true friend will hold you accountable and encourage you to meet your specific weight loss or exercise goals. You want to politely stay away from office workers who ask you out to happy hour if part of your plan is to cut back on the 3 hour drinking & eating binges that most happy hours promote. Even if that family member or friend does not exercise with you, the fact of telling them about your plan is great leverage for you to follow though and stick with it.

For many of you reading this book who don't yet see health as the most precious gift you'll ever receive in life, my hope is by the end of this book you'll decide to make a plan for some sort of regular exercise. Speaking of planning, if you look at most really successful celebrities, most of the highest paid business executives, and almost all world leaders, if you read their biographies, or have the opportunity to meet them in person, these people usually have a detailed plan for exercise. The last Pope had a plan to wake up at 5am every single morning (even Sundays) and do 30 minutes of exercise including 200 push-ups and sit-ups. Almost every President of the U.S. (who have less personal time than probably anybody on the planet as sometimes they have working dinners, conference calls, of overseas flights) make a plan to exercise every single day to boost their energy to allow them to work the 12+ hour days Presidents often do. I had the honor of meeting President G.W. Bush several times and his secret to his lean physique and his amazing energy was his daily exercise. President Bush would play a brisk game of tennis, walk, run, or lift weights, do something physical every single day, no matter how busy his schedule. Even President John F. Kennedy (who had serious health issues his entire life) scheduled exercise every single day to keep his health in check and to keep his energy levels up especially during the long hours and stress he endured during the Cuban Missile Crisis. Many "A-List" actors I've had the privilege of working with are often in the gym at 4 or 5am before they head to set for their extremely long workdays. If all of these movers and shakers (many of whom work 12 – 16 hours days) still manage to wake up by 5am, you should make a plan to fit some daily exercise into your schedule as well. Turn over a new leaf yourself and "work out like a President!".

No matter what level of health you're at, **the next chapter will outline a simple strategy to start exercising every day without any additional time or thought**. The concept of "NET" (No Extra Time) is a very powerful strategy I learned years ago from Tony Robbins and it is something you can start right now... even while you continue to read this book!

"Fresh air impoverishes the doctor."
- Danish Proverb

CHAPTER THIRTY-ONE (31):
No Time to Exercise? Try "NET" Time!

ALL legitimate health experts and doctors agree that **exercise is a critical part of good health** and that's why it is one of the 5 sections of this book. It is my deepest hope that even if you are not an "exercise buff", you will read this chapter and implement some of the strategies including the concept of "NET" time. NET time stands for "No Extra Time" and it will change your life if you apply the simple (yet profound) strategy introduced to me many years ago by Tony Robbins. There are dozens of reasons why people don't go to the gym, go running, bicycling, hiking, play sports, go work outdoors in the garden, etc., but most of them come down to the same excuse: "I just don't have time". In our modern day, busy world, time is our most precious commodity, so there is some validity to this excuse, but if you understand this concept of multi-tasking or doing several things (including exercise) at the same exact time, you'll be able to get exercise while doing another task in "No Extra Time"! A great example of this is the uber-efficient businessman and friend named Tom who has an hour long commute every morning. Instead of just driving and listening to talk radio and letting obnoxious drivers influence his state of mind every morning, Tom (an agent in Beverly Hills) utilizes NET time by making a short list of 3 or 4 important clients on the east coast he needs to speak with. While it's 8am on the west coast, it is 11am on the east coast (a great time for Tom to reach people on the phone before the lunch hour). With this short list of important calls and his blue-tooth head set in his ear, Tom dials away and spends that hour making these 3 or 4 (sometimes 5 or 6 important calls) before he even gets to his office. Now if you take this simple concept of NET time every day and do it with exercise, there is NO MORE EXCUSE for you NOT to EXERCISE EVERY SINGLE DAY! Below are just a few examples:

CURRENT TASK	"NET" OPPORTUNITY	"NET" SOLUTION	NOTES
Return important business calls.	Hour long commute while you are returning phone calls & exercising your arms.	Get a "hand-grip" or stress ball in your car to work out your hands & arms each day.	Even just 10 minutes on each hand is good exercise while you are driving.
Trips to the post office, bank, etc.	Most people have to do these errands!	Walk or bicycle to some of these local errands.	If you don't live within a mile of your city center & have to drive, park your car and walk between all your "local" errands.
Entering your office building every day.	You have to get to your office every day anyway!	Change your habit of taking the elevator or escalator and instead climb the stairs every time you enter or exit the building.	Even just 2 - 3 flights of stairs is exercise that you're not getting now. If your office is on a higher floor (like the 15th floor) walk the first 5 floors & take the elevator from floor 5 up to 15. Build up your endurance over time.
Going to the grocery store	Walking in and out of the store.	Instead of fighting to find a close parking spot, park at the very end or rear of the parking lot. A brisk 1-minute walk in & out will give you a boost of energy. If you don't really need a shopping cart, carry your 2 or	In addition to getting a quick boost of energy, you'll avoid the frustration of circling the parking lot 2 – 3 times, save time, and eliminate scratches & door dings on your car!

		3 bags out with you.	
Reading a lengthy business report.	Use this hour or two that you have to read & get exercise at the same time.	Hop on a stationary bike and get a nice workout the same time you are reading!	Most gyms have stationary bikes. There are also affordable models for home use as well starting at just $100.
Lunch hour.	Instead of sitting down for an hour after sitting in your cubicle for 3 – 4 hours, walk during your lunch hour!	Get outside & walk while eating a light snack, or take your phone & catch up on personal calls. Get a co-worker to join you & make it even more fun!	You can also practice your deep diaphramic breathing while walking to oxygenate your body. You'll be completely energized while your co-workers are lethargic!
Personal phone calls to return at home.	Instead of just sitting down to return phone calls after work, utilize NET time to make it fun!	Take your cordless or cell phone out to your Jacuzzi. The warm water & jets will give you a massage. If you don't have a Jacuzzi, run a hot bath & work our your upper or lower body with rubber exercise bands while making phone calls.	After your phone calls are all made, take an extra 15 minutes to just relax and unwind. Make this your "personal" NET time!
Read a lengthy book (for business or pleasure).	Get the book "on tape" or an MP3.	Instead of sitting motionless while you "read", enjoy all your books while you are walking &	You'll usually retain more of your book while stimulating your physiology vs. reading in a

		getting exercise.	passive state.
Brainstorm solutions to a problem.	Any time you face a Problem!	Go outside for a walk while looking for solutions to your problem.	In addition to changing your venue (you're not just sitting in your office), the fresh air & moving your body will help you find a solution more quickly.
Exercise & get Inspired.	While going for a run.	If you're going for a run or bike ride just for exercise, spend 10 – 15 minutes shouting out Incantations!	By repeating your incantations over and over while doing physical exercise, you will get inspired!
Watching your favorite TV show.	Instead of just being a couch potato, get your body moving!	You can either ride a stationary bike while watching your favorite 30 or 60-minute show, or do exercises and stretches during the commercial breaks.	BONUS: in addition to getting NET exercise, you'll most likely stop the bad practice of snacking for a solid hour while sitting on the couch!
Planning your day, week, etc.	Get out of your office and start walking!	By walking in the great outdoors, you'll often come up with fresh new ideas to plan tasks for the upcoming day or week while getting exercise.	Instead of writing your "To Do" list on pen & paper, dictate notes to a digital recorder or your smart phone while they're fresh. Finalize all notes when you get back to your office.

The very latest trend are these new "treadmill desks". Instead of having an expensive office chair for their employees to sit down for 8 hours each day, Salo (a financial trading company in Minnesota) has implemented a test of treadmills, which butt right up to their employee's desks where they can use their computer and talk on the phone. The employees plod along at a very slow pace (normally just 1 or 2 mph), and initial feedback is that the employees have great energy all day long, are more alert, and one employee even lost 25 pounds in the first few months! Talk about the epitome of NET time... these folks are getting great exercise all day long while doing their work.

These are just a few examples of how you can easily get exercise while doing other tasks in "No Extra Time". This principal will change your life and get your body moving in the direction of better health. If any of your family members or close friends ever tell you: "I just don't have any time to exercise", DON'T LET THEM MAKE EXCUSES! Introduce them to this concept of NET time and you can help them get healthier in "no extra time" as well!

"Sometimes I get the feeling the aspirin companies are sponsoring my headaches."
- V.L. Allineare

CHAPTER THIRTY-TWO (32):
How Parents Can Set an Example!

If you're a kid reading this, take a close look at your parents (or grandparents when you see them). If they are overweight and don't exude a lot of energy, my guess is that they either have a poor diet, or they don't have a really active lifestyle. They say that retired people who don't find another vocation or serious hobby often die within 10 years of retirement. A published study indicates men and women who retire early at age 55 have a significantly increased risk of death, as compared with those who retire at 65. In this research, death was almost twice as likely in the first 10 years after retirement at age 55 compared with those who continued working! [32-1]

My take on this staggering death statistic is two-fold. One reason for an early death is not having a "purpose" in life, but the other major reason that contributes to early death is lack of exercise and body movement after retirement. Exercise (even something as simple as daily walks) is obviously good for your body, helps keep the weight off by burning calories, and improves circulation & blood flow making you feel better. If your parents plop in front of the TV (aka: the "boob tube") for hours on end every night while eating snacks, drinking alcohol or sodas, etc., my guess is that they are not in the same physical shape and not nearly as energetic as Jack LaLanne was in his 90s! If you have any older family members who are lethargic, sick, or simply overweight, take a good look at them and understand that this does NOT need to be you! While genetics can be a health factor, genes and genetics play a smaller role in health than what was once thought. You can make intelligent choices like reading this book and sharing the information with people you love like your parents or grandparents! Even if you don't watch a lot of TV, if you spend your afternoons playing video games and most of your night in front of the computer, make a decision right now to: 1) cut down the time sitting in front of these screens and 2) if you have several hours of office work or homework which requires you to work on your computer, take a break at least every hour. Sitting motionless at your computer for 4 – 5 hours straight is absolutely INSANE! 3) take a tip from my friend Nathan Agin who works at his computer (whether writing, editing, reading e-mails) while standing. He hardly ever gets tired compared to when he used to sit at his computer and he now has excellent posture! Not only will sitting down for extended periods of time suck the energy out of you like a vampire, but this will lead to bad posture, a dependence on caffeinated energy drinks, and most likely poor nutritional snack foods which could lead to all sorts of problems down the road.

If you're a parent reading this book and you are a "couch potato", make a decision right NOW to not only start exercising to get your health back, but most importantly to set an example for your kids that they can use the rest of their lives. Going outdoors in the woods for a hike, playing catch, going for a bike ride, or even just going for a walk are all great ways for family members to connect while doing your bodies some good. My father who beat a nasty battle with lung cancer (thank God) is now 80 and is in great shape by eating a healthy diet, but also because he exercises every single day. Even in the middle of winter when it can get really cold and windy in New York city (some days even snowing or sleeting), he always makes it a point to ask the whole family who wants to take a walk. Even just a 20 - 30 minute walk is a great energy boost after a large Christmas dinner. Thank you Dad for always setting a great example!

"Always laugh when you can. It is cheap medicine."
- **Lord Byron**

CHAPTER THIRTY-THREE (33):
Exercise Will Make you Sleep Better

Are you like too many people who have trouble sleeping, or do you ever hear your co-workers complain about insomnia (the Latin word for getting "no sleep")? In addition to not having a late dinner or a late night snack of junk food or alcohol within an hour of going to bed (common sense not to overload your digestive system right before trying to go to sleep), there are a few tips to get a restful sleep. Despite 30% of the U.S. population having insomnia, and the 10 million people now addicted to prescription sleep aids, for many people there is a natural way to get a better night's sleep... exercise! [33-1]

Once you start exercising during the day (preferably in the morning), or if you start doing NET exercise during the day or afternoon, not only will you feel better, but you'll sleep better. Ever wonder why kids who are very active (running or biking around the neighborhood all day or playing lots of sports), usually fall asleep quickly? Since their bodies have been active all day long, bedtime is a chance for their bodies to finally rest and recover. If you are one of those people who sit in an office cubicle all day and then sit down in front of the TV for 3 or 4 hours each night, your body is not inclined to want to stay motionless for another 7 or 8 hours in bed! However, if you work a full day including a good amount of exercise and body movement, your body will yearn to lie motionless at night as a way to rest. For many people who have a lot of stress or anxiety, exercise is a great way to help relieve this stress and therefore also help you sleep better. Here are a few tips (you may already know some of these), on how to get a better night's sleep:

1) Get some aerobic exercise during the day (preferably morning, NOT close to your bedtime).

2) Don't eat a late meal or snack within 2 hours of going to bed.

3) Don't drink lots of fluids right before bed (especially alcohol).

4) Cut out the "negative" TV right before bed (ex. nightly news, horror movies, etc.).

5) Do your best not to think about work or life's problems right before turning off the light. It's much better to read an inspiring book, magazine article or think about your goals & dreams.

6) Set a second alarm clock as a "back up" (I have three and one of them even has a battery back-up). This will completely put your mind at rest about waking up on time.

7) Leave a note pad by your bedside. If you think of something important that you need to handle the next day, you can roll over, write a note, and NOT worry about it. This process will clear your mind completely!

8) Retire and wake up at approximately the same time each night & day.

9) Think about 1 or 2 things you are grateful for (or could be) in your life right before you go to sleep.

This last one might be hard, especially if you just lost your job (like many folks these days), are about to lose your house, are getting sued, or perhaps just lost a loved one. But if you keep asking: "What could I possibly be grateful for?" your mind will eventually come up with 1 or 2 things that you can feel grateful for.

Most people can function perfectly with 5 – 8 hours of sleep. Many people need just 6 or 7. However you NEED to master the art of getting a good night's sleep rather than not addressing this issue which can affect your whole life when you are "awake" (or struggling to stay awake). Besides the obvious insomnia problems (thousands of work related work accidents and car crashes that occur each year), being tired is no way to live your life. In addition to the other tips, the # 1 way to improve your sleep pattern at night and boost your energy during the day is proper exercise! As the Nike slogan says: "Just Do It!"

⇔ SUBSTITUTE: The next time you're thinking about reaching for a sugar-loaded snack or a coffee for a quick pick me up, get out of the house and take a short walk. Even if it is really cold or snowing out, dress warmly and the act of walking in the fresh air will not only energize you, but will also warm you up and boost your metabolism!

SECTION V:
FAITH

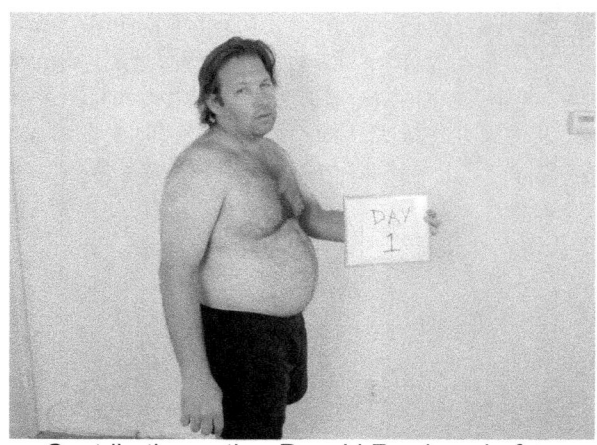

Contributing author Ronald Farnham before
doing an "Alkalize & Energize" cleanse.

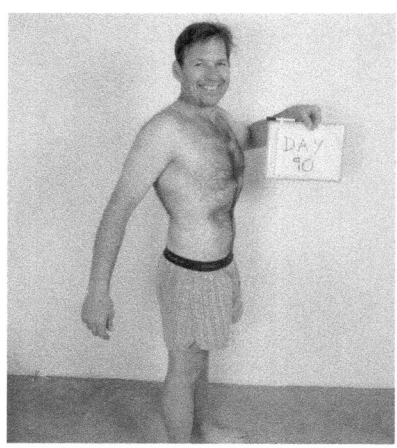

Ronald felt so amazing after 7 days he continued.
Here's the "new" Ronald 90 days later and 60 lbs. lighter!

CHAPTER THIRTY-FOUR (34):
Notice the Happy
as Well as the Depressed People

This last section of this book is very broad and I decided to title it "Faith" which may represent different things to different people. In terms of excellent health, energy, and overall happiness, some sort of faith (belief, outlook, or whatever you want to label it) is absolutely critical. This doesn't mean you have to be religious (although for many people religion is an important part of their lives), but you must believe in a higher power or something spiritual including the fact that YOU can control your beliefs as to how you live your life. Many circumstances are beyond our control, and I firmly believe that the "meaning" of things that happen to us in life is largely determined by your interpretation of events. For example: two people could get in the same type of car accident on the same exact stretch of road and those two people could have completely different experiences based upon their "meaning" or "interpretation" of that accident. One person could walk away smiling and be totally grateful that he or she had no major injuries, nobody else involved in the accident was killed or injured, and that person will walk away with a new meaning of their life ahead of them. Another person might look at the same accident and start swearing and cussing because he or she has scratches and some major dents in their car and are now late for an important meeting. Instead of feeling grateful, this person is focused on all the negatives including dealing with the insurance company, etc. This "faith" all starts with you taking some control of your mind (along with your health, since there is without a doubt a mind-body connection). I applaud you taking the initiative and the fact that you have this book in your hands right now. If you didn't have any faith (or some sort of belief) that you can control certain aspects of your health, you probably wouldn't have purchased this book.

Before we delve further into the "Faith" section, think of a person in your life (this could be a friend, relative, or acquaintance) who always seems happy, believes that life is a gift, and that life every day despite occasional challenges is great. Observe this optimistic, sunny person for a few days find out if this positive role model:

1) Watches a lot of television including the news (more than 3 hours a day)?

2) Hangs around with negative people most of the time?

3) Works at a job that they can't stand?

4) Has any kind of drug or alcohol problem?

Common sense would say of course not! This optimistic, fun-loving person does not necessarily have to have faith, or believe in God (this section is not meant to be religious in any particular sect), but my guess is your friend has an underlying "faith" in the positive forces of life and nature in general including a "glass ½ full" view as opposed to a "glass ½ empty" outlook on life. If you really observe your auspicious friend, his or her attitude is mostly a mind-set. People are not necessarily born to be pessimists or optimists, but through a series of habits including how they focus their time, attention, and thoughts will have different outlooks on life. A great example of this is the majority of Americans who wake up every morning and first thing they do is turn on their televisions. Every single morning, millions of Americans get bombarded with news on the television, and later on the radio for those who commute to work. It's understandable to see how many people have a negative point of view of "how bad" things are in the world. Now I'm not suggesting you never watch or listen to the news, but **if all you do is program your mind each morning with negative, depressing, and sometimes politically distorted news**, this is NOT healthy. By focusing your attention on natural disasters, wars, unemployment, the banking crisis, our failing schools, unemployment, local murders in your town, another huge oil spill, rising gas prices, political scandals, bank robberies, the current health epidemic, the national debt of our country as well as other floundering economies around the world, etc., **this is an INSANE way to start your day**

with the right mindset! Here are a few statistics for you to ponder: The January 2007 publication "Lawyers and Settlements" reported that the U.S. market for antidepressants accounted for 66% of the entire global market vs. 23% in Europe & 11% for the rest of the world. [34-1] 66% of consumption of the world's antidepressant medication by a single country is insane! We should learn a lesson from the Fijians who are considered by many to be the happiest people in the world. Fiji is far from the richest country in the world, but the Fijian people are doing many of tips mentioned in this book and are consistently happy. Here's another jaw dropping statistic: from 1988–2008, the rate of antidepressant use in the United States among all ages increased nearly 400%! [34-2] This included the exponential growth market in teenage antidepressants with the study including those children and teens 12 – 17 years old. In 1985 sales of antidepressants in the U.S. were just $240 million, in 2004 sales were an astounding $11.2 billion, with some people estimating that the revenues for antidepressants in the US could surpass $15 billion in a few short years!

Common sense would dictate that taking pills is not always the answer. There are a few easy techniques (as long as you follow them) to become a positive person who has faith. My friend Monroe Mann has been in the entertainment business for many years and is one of the very few who has survived the incredible challenges to get scripts completed, raised financing for films (outside of the studio system), and actually got movies distributed. Monroe is focused like a laser on his outcomes by always asking empowering questions including: "How can I achieve this result?". The other trait Monroe has that I admire is he is ALWAYS positive and incredibly optimistic (you have to be when raising money for films, writing an award-winning script, or when trying to get films picked up for distribution these days). I've never heard Monroe use words like "can't" or "impossible". They simply are not in his vocabulary. As mentioned, there are very consistent patterns for people being optimistic and getting things done, just as there are specific patterns for getting depressed! In the next few chapters we'll study some more specific causes of depression, look at some suggestions and solutions to become more positive, and I'll share some shining examples from some other positive friends. I'll also share some insights into a brave hero named Witold Pilecki, who witnessed hundreds of his close friends get murdered over the course of 4 years. People starved, tortured, and murdered right before his very eyes on a daily basis! Keep reading on how Witold stayed the course, remaining an eternal optimist through his unwavering faith!

"We cannot continue.
Our pension costs and health care costs
for our employees are going to bankrupt this city."
- New York Mayor Michael Bloomberg

CHAPTER THIRTY-FIVE (35):
Current Programing ...Have You Lost Faith?

Have you noticed that the vast majority of people today do not have as much belief (faith) in our government, our schools, our economy, our future generation, and our future in general as most people did just 20 years ago? Two years I made my annual trip back to New Jersey to visit my mother and the rest of the family for Christmas. Although I communicate with my mother via the phone, email, etc. on a regular basis, this was the first time I had seen her in person in almost a year. I noticed that she looked a little older (you often notice changes of people if there's been a time lapse), but what was the most shocking to me was that while she still had faith in God, she had lost faith in almost everything and everybody else and was not as cheerful and upbeat as she usually was (part of this was related to health issues which can sap the energy out of anyone). The first day I got home, I noticed she was worried sick about the "worst recession ever", the "bank crisis", the "horrific wars", the "crumbling education system", etc. After visiting her for about a week and being immersed in her environment, I figured out the problem was the bad "programming" that she was installing in her mind every single day. This was her ritual most mornings:

1) Get out of bed early in the morning (often it would be dark) as my Mom is usually an early riser. Like most people, my mother has a standard clock radio with an alarm that is not the most pleasant sound to wake up to.

2) Turn on the television to watch and listen to all the news.

3) Go downstairs and get a cup of coffee.

4) Turn on one of the talk radio shows. Normally around the holidays, a large portion of these shows are ranting about politics with the recent elections and current events including the wars in Afghanistan & Iraq.

5) A while later while making breakfast, she would watch the morning news switching back and forth between different networks. It doesn't matter which news channel you watch (national or local), MOST of the news is extremely negative taking about the latest Wall Street scandal, the most recent U.S. corporation to file bankruptcy, the tens of thousands of manufacturing jobs that were just lost, the skyrocketing foreclosure rates, the local war hero who just committed suicide yesterday, the obesity epidemic, and the exponential growth of ADD and ADHD of our kids who are attending the growing number of failing schools. The most positive story might be a warning to make sure you don't eat any of the local vegetables, which could be tainted by Salmonela or a report to be careful about the rising toxicity in the local water supply!

6) Then as my mom would be getting ready to enjoy her breakfast, she would start reading the local newspaper, which had awful headlines covering the local politician who just got caught cheating on his wife with a prostitute while embezzling funds from a local charity.

7) Of course the back section of the paper has the obituaries, which was a must read section even if she didn't know any of the people who passed away that day.

This all transpired in the first two hours of each day! What kind of state do you think all of this left my mother (or anyone else for that matter)?

This quick story I share is in no way to pick on my mother, as I used to have similar habits many years ago and I was not a very optimistic or sunny person in the morning. In fact, I really didn't really get "on a roll" until lunchtime when I used to go for a plate of barbeque chicken wings, curly French fries, and free refills of Coke with my good friend Bill Barnes. After some good old-fashioned barbeque and a few large cokes, Bill and I would be ready to hit the phones for the rest of the day calling our customers when we both worked at Xerox. Bill was an awesome guy who I miss dearly, since a few years ago he also died from cancer. Being great friends with Bill and seeing the grief on his wife's face at his funeral and the sadness his young daughter went through was awful. This was one of the first wake up calls that I should start eating a healthier diet.

Anyway, getting back to the story of my mother, does this sound familiar? Like somebody YOU know very well? This "programming" that too many of us have as an everyday habit might not be the best WAY TO START YOUR DAY! Another example from my Xerox days was a co-worker who would stop by my cubicle each morning around 9:00am and recite 2 or 3 horrific stories from the morning news. This would often be a 5 minute rant (sometimes it would last longer), where he would bring up some grisly murder or some other horrific story, and before you knew it 3 or 4 other co-workers would chime in and add their 2 cents worth. While this co-worker was a friend (who meant well), he was probably one of the most negative guys around. I have to believe part of that was caused by reciting the negative news stories each morning. Remember that the more shocking, controversial, and horrific the headlines are each day, the more newspapers are sold, and the more viewers go on-line. But being too immersed in these negative stories is NOT the best "faith" to have. What I love about getting news now from the internet is you can pick and choose what stories you want to read quickly without having to sit through all the other negative news stories. Being informed each day, doesn't have to mean losing your faith!

CHAPTER THIRTY-SIX (36):
Reignite the Power of Faith... Believe it!

It's important to note that nearly 1,200 studies have been conducted on how prayer and faith improves health. Harvard scientist Dr. Herbert Benson found it initiates a relaxation response in which heart rate, breathing, and metabolism slow down promoting healing and boosting your immune system. [36-1] So how does one reignite faith? How do you start believing in all that is good and begin to have a more optimistic view of life? In addition to faith in God, Allah, a divine spirit, or perhaps the Universe, or mankind in general (whoever and whatever you believe in), what you continually choose to focus on determines your beliefs and will impact the quality of your entire life. Your perception of today's society, our government, our politicians, our teachers, our schools, our neighbors, etc. and how it affects your life is greatly determined by how you program your mind. Are you one of the MANY people in the U.S. who go through the same ritual of bombarding themselves with news first thing in the morning? Tony Robbins has a great saying that you should: "See things as they are, but not worse than they are". While these are challenging times and I don't want to minimize the impact this temporary recession has had on people's lives, in reality the 8 – 9% unemployment is nowhere near as bad as the 25% unemployment during in the great depression. The banking crisis of today can not be compared to the 1930s where many of the major banks completely failed (there was no government bailout to save the banks), and every week dozens of bankers and Wall Street executives committed suicide by jumping out of high rise buildings in Manhattan! While it is tragic that we've lost over 4,400 U.S. soldiers in Iraq to date over the past 10 years (and my heart goes out to any friends or relatives who have lost comrades in battle or just being in the field), think about how many more families and loved ones were affected during Vietnam where the U.S. lost 58,209 brave souls, or after World War II which ended up with 405,399 U.S. casualties! If you look at the horrible news broadcasts or the printed news every day (most of the headlines are sensationalized to sell papers or "hook" you to watch their morning news show vs. another news channel), one might think that Iran is weeks away from finalizing their arsenal of nuclear weapons and at that point will launch a fleet of missiles to destroy the entire country of Israel and therefore starting World War III in the very near future! I certainly don't want to downplay the tension and problems in the Middle East right now, but focusing on that every single morning before you leave for work is not solving the problem, and NOT putting you in the best state for a productive day.

So how specifically can you regain faith and have a positive outlook every day? It all starts with **Questions**. Yes... simple questions you ask yourself (consciously or unconsciously) every single day. If your alarm clock goes off early in the morning and you are hung-over, or have an upset stomach from too much food the night before, you're first question each day might be: "Ahhhhh.... Why me?". You should go back and re-read Section I on alkalinity. Starting the day with any alcohol, toxins, or excess acids in your system is not the best way to start your day with lots of energy and excitement. Assuming you got a good night's sleep (at least 5 – 7 hours), the first question you should ask yourself is NOT: "Oh God, why do I have to get up now?". If you are really healthy and have excellent energy, you shouldn't have to hit the snooze button only to have the alarm screech in your ear again 15 minutes later. If you are in that situation, perhaps you then ask yourself: "Oh, please can I just have 15 more minutes of rest?" If you focus on what you have, instead of what you don't have (like the extra 15 minutes of sleep you wish for), that focus can change your whole outlook for the day. I have a sister who recently lost one of her fingers to an infection, I had a cousin who lost use of her entire arm to gout (eventually cancer spread throughout her whole body and she died), I have a few friends in wheelchairs who will never walk again for the rest of their lives. Each day when I get up I think about what I HAVE (including 10 fingers and 10 toes that still function perfectly). I say a quick "thank you" that I still have all my limbs and can get out of bed and walk every day. Coming from that mind-set of what "I HAVE" vs. what "I don't have" yet (a Tesla electric car in case you are wondering), is a much healthier outlook! A better morning question I now ask every day is: "What am I grateful for today?". That will usually generate several quick answers like feeling grateful for my hands and feet that work perfectly (unlike many older relatives who have arthritis or joint pains). Another positive answer I get when I ask the same question is: "I am so grateful that I have a roof over my head, electricity, and hot water". This is quite a contrast to almost a almost dozen homeless people I now see sleeping in their cars around North Hollywood and Studio City. Some of these people are (or were) professional white-collar types who perhaps lost their home to foreclosure when they lost their jobs with all the recent layoffs. Having electricity and water 24 hours a day is something we take for granted, yet tens of millions of people around the world either have no electricity (or sporadic) or clean running water that is drinkable. So by asking the right questions each morning, I feel a sense of gratitude for what I DO HAVE in my life. Another great question to ask in the morning is; "What am I happy about in my life right now?". If your brain freezes up and it answers back: "Nothing", perhaps you could ask a better follow up question: "What COULD you be happy about right now?". Perhaps one of your relatives recently beat cancer and is still alive? Perhaps you are one of the few people in your department who did not get downsized and still has a job? Thinking about the things that you HAVE in your life will make you feel more grateful and help you start the day in a much more positive, optimistic state. The question I asked myself this morning is: "How did I get so lucky that I have the right to vote?" This is an empowering question to ask in an age where hundreds of millions of people around the world don't have true voting rights, and tens of millions of women and minorities in some countries have no vote. I really appreciate the rights I have today. I sometimes think about the brave men and women who fought and died for rights like this, which we now have in this country. There is a saying from Tony Robbins I always remember whenever I face what seem to be insurmountable challenges. Tony often says: "Your biggest problem is someone else's dream." No matter how bad your finances are, or how bad things might be if you just lost a loved one, there are 27 million people right now around the world wrongfully imprisoned or working as slaves! As mentioned, there are millions of people in 3rd world countries who don't have clean drinking water or enough food to keep them healthy. There are scores of people in Syria every single day who lose loved ones (sometimes their entire family without warning) right in front of their eyes in the heat of battle. There are tens of millions of kids around the world who never get the opportunity to attend college, let alone the equivalent of a high school education which so many of us in the U.S. take for granted. When you change your perspective for a moment and really think about the opportunities most of us have, we are very lucky. If things still seem really bad, and you can't seem to find any faith to get through an extremely challenging situation another empowering question I ask myself is: "What will this situation (problem, incident) mean to me 10 years from now?" That is a powerful question to ask and gets you looking at the "Big" picture of life and helps you refocus on what is really important in your life and regain your faith! Most big problems at this very moment might seem huge, but in the course of your lifetime, do not mean that much, so there's no point in worrying yourself sick about something you might not be able to impact or change anyway!

By asking better questions each morning, you CAN control your focus and your emotions to reignite your faith to become one of those "optimistic, positive" people you probably already know. However I do have one important warning. This does NOT mean every single day is going to be perfect (that would make life boring anyway). You're not going to be cheery and feel fantastic every single day (life always has its ups and downs). From time to time we all have incredible challenges and obstacles we face that can actually make us stronger. So take these setbacks with a grain of salt and remember there is always tomorrow. I promise you if you keep asking better (empowering, positive) questions, you will always end up better off than you were, and have a better outlook on life along the way.

We already discussed in Section IV that simply moving your body through exercise (changing your physiology) will immediately change your state. To recap here in this chapter, you can also change your focus (your whole outlook on life) by asking better questions! I have a question for you...Are you ready to implement this simple strategy right now or at least tomorrow morning? The answer is up to YOU.

"Health is like money, we never have a true idea of its value until we lose it."
- **Josh Billings**

CHAPTER THIRTY-SEVEN (37):
Stories & Examples of Extremely Positive People

In addition to exercise (changing your physiology), and asking yourself better questions (changing your focus), there is another specific and important way to change your state to feel great. This simple tip is to change your VOCABULARY.

One of my best friends in college was Tony Knight. The very first day I met Tony (we both had an interest in waterskiing and he at the time was a nationally ranked tournament skier), I was taken by his huge smile and firm handshake. In addition, there seemed to be an energy (or aura) about him that just made you feel great. If you ask the question in your office, at school (or even at a social setting): "How are you doing?". I bet that 75% of the people would say: "OK", "Hanging in there", "Not so bad", "Getting by", "Paying my dues to the man", "Keeping the old lady off my back", or some other answer. These are NOT the most positive or empowering responses! EVERY single time during my 4 years at college (and ever since then when I do see Tony), if anybody asked Tony how he was doing, he would immediately respond with: "FANTASTIC! ...how are you doing?". He didn't yell it in an obnoxious way, but he really was feeling fantastic in a genuine way and wanted to know how you were doing. The only time I ever heard Tony change his vocabulary and respond with a different word when asked how he was, were the few times when he responded: "AWESOME! ...how are you?". Tony seemed to have everything going for him. He had excellent grades, he was a nationally ranked water-skier, had a beautiful girlfriend, had lots of friends everywhere he went, drove a really cool 4 x 4 Jeep, and yet not one single person on campus was jealous of him, or could ever say a single negative word about him. By instilling a "positive" vocabulary into his daily lifestyle, Tony was always in a positive state. Even when his Jeep broke down one time and we were stranded on the side of the road, instead of getting upset or frustrated, he simply remarked: "Darn it... this means one less beer we'll get to drink at the party tonight!" Tony always focused on solutions rather than the problem, which is anther great quality to have. Here is another example of an incredible person who changed his state through vocabulary.

In the 1940s there was a Jewish gentleman named Witold Pilecki who after the German occupation of Poland walked into a German SS roundup and volunteered to be a prisoner! That was NOT a typo. Captain Pilecki literally volunteered to be taken to one of the worst concentration camps where hundreds of his friends died every year. His work duty (at that camp and other concentration camps he was moved to) included carting off thousands of dead to burial pits, or witnessing thousands of people in his camp march towards the gas chambers every day only to exit though smoke and ashes through the towering black chimneys. He noticed that his friends who froze to death, starved, or died of disease often had a bad vocabulary where they would be chanting to themselves what a "living hell" they were in, or "how miserable" they were in the "awful conditions". Wiltold had a clear mission to break out of the camp and to help others break out, and both subliminally and verbally he instilled his own language (a "positive" vocabulary). When he woke up each morning he would tell himself: "I am one of the lucky ones to be alive!". When others were falling down from sickness on work duty, he would tell himself that he was "healthy" and "strong". I have to believe that his positive vocabulary and faith helped him be one of the few members in his group who made it out alive! [37-1] Another Holocost survivor (and an author as well) was Viktor Frankl who as a psychiatrist understood how language and vocabulary could help change people's states, and just like Wiltold Pilecki, Viktor was also one of the lucky ones who made it out alive and ended up publishing several excellent books including my favorite Man's Search for Meaning.

Another stellar example of how vocabulary can change your state is my good friend Monroe Mann whom I consider a modern day Renaissance man. Monroe is a best selling author, an entertainment attorney, performance coach, strategist, consultant, publicist, marketing expert, talented musician, award-winning actor, film director, and a film producer. I'm sure I left a few things out, but you get the picture that this guy is no slacker! I always observe Monroe's vocabulary whether he's e-mailing me at 5am, or we're talking on the phone at midnight. Monroe uses words like "Excellent", "Powerful" "Unstoppable", "Amazing" and my favorite "Romp-On!". I've never heard Monroe speak a negative word and he rarely uses words that don't have some kind of emotion behind them.

Another quick example of vocabulary impacting someone's state and energy is another good friend Crystal. I've known Crystal for several years and she is a sweet heart and a very hard worker. She often works 10, 11, or 12 hour days, and her work can be very stressful with clients who put demanding deadlines on her. She often does not leave the office until 8 or 9pm and very often when we talk on the phone, I will ask her how her day was and how she is doing. Crystal will almost always answer: "Oh... I'm very tired." She might use the word "tired" 2 or 3 different times in our conversation and put major emphasis on that one word. Now there are times we all get "tired", I often do after a 12 or 13 hour workday which are common on film sets. Sometimes the lack of energy is from metal activity, other times it might be physical, (we've already discussed how acid food & sugar will make you tired so we won't discuss that here), but whatever the cause, it is NOT helpful to be repeating to yourself either subliminally (or aloud) that you are "tired". The more you mention it and tell others how "tired" you feel, will only make you feel more "tired". If you truly have an exhausting day (I've had a few 16 & 17 hours work days where it was a challenge to keep my eyelids open), I've been able to get an energy boost by changing my vocabulary. If someone asks on set how I'm doing after a 16 hour day, I'll make a joke about it and answer in my best Arnold Schwarzenegger imitation: "Like the terminator... I'm unstoppable!" or I might respond: "Never felt better!" Not only do I believe that saying something positive helps boost your energy, but it also changes the state of others around you and often gets a laugh, which also generates some positive energy in the room.

The legendary Joel Osteen said recently: "Be positive or be quiet!" as he has witnessed hundreds of people in his church live more positive, healthy lives including several cancer survivors who spoke positive words out loud to help them heal. I could go on and on about examples of people who have positive vocabulary and others (usually by accident or habit) have a disempowering vocabulary, but the test for YOU is to see what specific impact vocabulary and words have on your state. The first step for you is to observe one of your friends, co-workers, or family members for just a few hours. Write down notes or make a mental observation of all the key words and what "vocabulary" they are using. If they are using negative words, are they themselves a little down, or not that fun to be around? If they are using words that have no positive emotion, are these people boring or not the most exciting? If you have friends who repeat a certain word over and over again such as: "stressed" or "overwhelmed", do those friends always seemed overwhelmed when you see them? By contrast do you have a family member or friend who uses a specific empowering word like "fun" or "enjoyable"? When you see or talk to this person on the phone, does he or she seem in good spirits? If you can't find a family member or friend who uses positive vocabulary on a regular basis, my challenge to you is find someone. See if you can find someone who only uses positive vocabulary such as my film producing partner and good friend Cam MacGregor who uses fun, dynamic words such as "fabulous", "stupendous", and "amazing". Every time I see Cam, he has a smile on his face and he has this positive energy that makes him fun to be around. Learn from your own experience and then TAKE ACTION yourself to instill your own positive vocabulary. Once you install a few empowering words (whatever words you choose), after just 3 or 4 days, you'll be amazed with the results, as will any friends or family members you encounter. They just might find you to be a "fun loving, energetic" person!

CHAPTER THIRTY-EIGHT (38):
The Internal Drugs Your Body
<u>Manufactures for Free!</u>

The U.S. now has over 150 million people taking prescription drugs on a regular basis and that doesn't begin to include all the over the counter (OTC) medications many of which were available by prescription just a few years ago. A fast growing segment for prescription drugs is the millions of kids now on ADD, ADHD, & ADHT medications! In fact there are rumors going on in the psychiatric medical community that next year the FDA will approve a liquid form ADHD medication. This will make it easier for millions of new young kids who can't take pills to start drinking banana and cherry flavored ADHD medicine just as easy as cough syrup. With the continuing expansion of new medicines and the exponential growth of people in the U.S. now taking prescriptions (including kids and teens) is not good for the health of our country, and also unsustainable to our economy! Is there a solution to this epidemic or any light at the end of the tunnel? Yes there is, if you understand that in most cases, there are natural alternatives (actual natural hormones and chemicals) that your body can manufacture and deliver for free! You might know Dr. Deepak Choprah from the 65 books he has written (many are best sellers), and in addition to being a prolific writer, Chopra taught at the medical schools of Tufts University, Boston University and Harvard University. He later became Chief of Staff at the New England Memorial Hospital before establishing a private practice. In his books the consistent message Dr. Choprah delivers and the advice he gives to patients is to understand through meditation, focus, and positive thoughts, your endocrine glands can often produce the equivalent prescriptions in "your own body's internal pharmacy" vs. having to buy store bought drugs. Your internal all-natural hormones such as adrenaline, cortisol and others can be just as effective as an expensive prescription purchased at your local CVS drug store or Walgreen's pharmacy for zero cost. A great example is the hormone oxytocin that acts primarily as a neuromodulator in the brain and is best known its roles in sexual reproduction in females, in particular during and after childbirth. It is released in large amounts after distension of the cervix and uterus during labor, facilitating birth.

Robert E. Battmer, M.D. (a gynecology physician & surgeon) comments: "We simply need to follow nature's plan to replace diminishing hormones with natural hormones that we've known about for nearly five decades. It is all very safe. The benefits are numerous and dramatic:

1) Human hormones do not cause cancer, they prevent it.

2) Heart and vascular disease is prevented.

3) Aging of cells is significantly slowed.

4) Osteoporosis is prevented or even reversed.

5) Mental and/or emotional dysfunction is prevented or reversed.

6) Anti-depressant drugs are frequently rendered unnecessary or the dosage can be lowered." [38-1]

Unlocking your internal pharmacy starts with "positive" emotions including but not limited to: love (by the far the most powerful), humor, optimism, and hope. Triggers can include: nature, pets, playing, music, movies, poetry, and hobbies that you are passionate or excited about. There are thousands of case studies that have been done with laughter especially in patients by Dr. Norman Cousins who has been called the father of laughter therapy medicine. In fact Dr. Cousins treated his own pain from many ailments including his life-threatening joint disease with a 10-minute daily dose of laughter.

The advanced stage of using positive vocabulary (you read about in the last chapter) is using "affirmations" where you repeat positive, meaningful phrases over and over. If you take a phrase and put lots of emotion behind it and coordinate a power gesture or physical body movement to that phrase, these are called "Incantations" which can CHANGE YOUR LIFE forever. I believe one of the reasons, I've been lucky enough to have such excellent health (in addition to alkalizing, hydrating, oxygenating, and exercising) is that I've also done my own incantation at least a dozen times every single day for the last 5 years: "I AM SO GRATEFUL FOR MY PERFECT HEALTH!" I shout this out when I'm running in the morning or exercising, or sometimes when driving my car." If I get stuck in traffic and someone in the car next to me sees me doing this incantation, they probably think I'm yelling at someone on the phone, since most everybody talks hands free these days when driving. Here's an important note: I don't feel perfect 365 days a year as the human body goes through cycles of health, sickness, low energy, high energy, etc., but as I repeat my incantation every day being grateful for my perfect health, signals are sent to my brain and throughout the rest of my body that I am in perfect health. This is a hard concept to grasp at first, but ask any M.D. or therapist about incantations and they will confirm what powerful tools they can be. In fact, it has been scientifically proven that repeated incantations change your physiology, and have even helped cancer patients recover. Make up your own incantation such as: "I'm so grateful for the unwanted pounds I'm shedding every day on the way to great health!", "I'm a lean, mean fighting machine!", or "My heart is getting stronger and my health is getting better every single day!". Many cancer survivors, people who have made it out of P.O.W. camps, top sales people, millionaires, inventors, and truly successful innovators and entrepreneurs all claim that daily incantations gave them faith and turned their lives around to levels most other people could only dream about. I could tell you dozens of stories of people who've used empowering vocabulary and incantations to save their lives and turn other people's lives around. The first is Tony Robbins who had a freak growth spurt due to an imbalanced Pituitary gland. This critical gland (which controls growth) got so out of control that Tony shot up over 1 foot in height in a single year! A few years later when Tony was having some problems, several doctors were so worried upon doing a brain scan, that they wanted to do brain surgery right away. Luckily Tony opted NOT to rush into surgery and turned his life around (I'm convinced partly due to his daily incantations) and he's had no major gland problems for over 25 years. Another great story is legendary singer Naomi Judd who was diagnosed many years ago by physicians that she had Hepatitis C and was given less than 3 years to live! Through her empowering vocabulary and her positive attitude, she not only survived but many years later Naomi remarks: "I am a medically documented miracle." [38-2] If you have any doubt that your body can manufacture chemicals that can improve your health or for that matter keep you alive all you have to do is ask any physician, psychiatrist, or coroner what month do most older, sick people die? The answer is January. Why? Because most really old people (let's say in their 90s or 100+ especially) get to the point where life is getting to be a struggle, or they are immobile, partially blind, crippled, etc. These people have faith and can energize their body to fight through one final Thanksgiving, one final Christmas (to be with loved ones), but come January 1st they see another entire year of struggle ahead and they often lose their will in January and that is the month most of these people quietly pass away. Part of faith is having something to look "forward" to.

What I respect about Dr. Choprah, Dr. Battmer, Dr. Cousins, and a few other well known physicians is while they still believe in the power of medicines and surgery when needed, they are promoting the plethora of options to let the body heal itself which under ideal circumstances (with an excellent diet, enough exercise, and proper rest) works wonders. It's common sense that if all the other animals in the world can heal themselves without synthetic or prescription drugs, you should be able to heal yourself as well with your own internal drugs that your body manufactures for free!

CHAPTER THIRTY-NINE (39):
The Bad Drugs Your Body Manufactures

You don't need a medical background to know that stress (or any kind of worrying) creates acid, which can lead to ulcers, heartburn, etc. If serious, stress can lead to massive health problems including high blood pressure and even heart attacks. Stress hormones such as cortisol and norepinephrine are released by the body in situations that are interpreted as being potentially dangerous, and in the rare situation that there is danger, these hormones are released to alert the body to avoid danger, and of course this can be a good thing. However just as your internal biological pharmacy manufactures "good" drugs, these acidic "bad" drugs in your system can wreck havoc to your health. When you don't have "faith" and are thinking negative (vs. positive and pleasant) thoughts, your mind and body can fall into the trap of depression, lack of focus, and hypertension. Your body's stress hormones can rob your body's energy supplies, which is why stressed out, negative people are often fatigued. These "bad" drugs can also affect your heart rate, blood pressure, breathing rate and even shut down metabolic processes such as digestion, reproduction, growth and immunity. A decrease in testosterone levels in males and irregular menstrual cycles in females can also occur, as well as increased likelihood of infectious diseases, illnesses, and cancer. This is why students who are under a severe amount of stress during final exam week (in combination with very little sleep) often get sick. To counteract the release of these bad drugs (hormones which are released in your body), yoga and meditation can really help as well as any of the exercises we discussed in the previous section. Remember there is a very real mind-body connection, so with a little discipline and focus, you can help eliminate or minimize these "bad" drugs from being manufactured in your body in the first place.

CHAPTER FORTY (40): The Tide is Turning!

Despite the doom & gloom I witnessed at the last few Medco events and Health Benefit fairs, there are a few people and a few schools now making a positive difference. I believe the most profound change for our future needs to start with the younger generation and our kids BEFORE more and more of them get diabetes, get hooked on ADHD medication, miss out on their childhood potential due to obesity, develop heart disease, or get cancer. Here are three (3) exciting examples of schools and students who are making a difference:

1. The first is a top-notch elementary school in Morristown, NJ called The Peck School. I saw a picture of the graduating class of 2012 and was shocked not to see a single OBESE kid...not one! Now in all fairness, there might have been one or two kids in the back rows of the photo who had a few extra pounds, but I figured this modern miracle needed further investigation. After looking at the photograph with a magnifying loop and later calling the school, I confirmed that the entire graduating class of The Peck School was in good shape and healthy! In addition to scheduled daily recesses, the real secret was in 2008, Peck School created an organic garden on campus where the students help grow their own vegetables, herbs, etc. which they use to feed themselves. The school also hired a company called Sage Dining, which has a very clear nutrition policy for healthy lifestyles and registered dieticians who vet every single meal served to these students! All the food grown from the garden helps offset some of the higher costs of feeding all the kids, faculty, and staff healthy, balanced, nutritious meals. What a brilliant concept... feeding our future kids great meals as they are in the classrooms for 8 hours each day to learn. Compared to many other schools which feed their kids "pink slime", French fries, and sodas or allowing Taco Bell or Pizza Hut to be approved food vendors, Peck School certainly deserves a Gold Star!

2. The second shining example is Oak Park High School in Southern California where I was privileged to screen our

new documentary film: "*What is the Electric Car?*". I knew it was a progressive school after the film screened when I asked people in the audience (both kids and their parents) to raise their hands if they drove an electric car to the school that night? About 15 people out of 150 people raised their hands! I was pleasantly surprised since the film was just rolling out in 2012 the same time when car dealerships were just starting to get a very limited supply of electric cars! Anyway, what also struck me looking out at the audience was that almost ALL the kids were in perfect shape, attentive, extremely intelligent, and simply looked really healthy. It turns out that the Oak Park Unified School District takes their student's food and nutrition VERY seriously! I later attended a function where the school had catered an event and almost all the hors d'oeuvres and entrees were organic vegetables & fruits along with tofu, beans, & sprout dishes along with healthy, homemade desserts. I did not see any dairy or meat served. I later spoke to Anthony Knight (the superintendent for the entire school district) and he confirmed how serious they were about the kid's nutrition for several reasons including health and well being of the students, as well as creating the best environment for students to learn and excel in their studies and athletics. Once again, what a brilliant concept! Now here's the real kicker... their school district in addition to serving organic food, has designated every Monday as "Meatless Mondays"! I asked how many students or parents complained about this and how many lawsuits the school had gotten from parents, board members, or trustees who were upset about taking the student's meat option away and he said NONE! I don't think this concept for "Meatless Mondays" would have worked 5 years ago, but with all the new research and studies linking meat and dairy to increased colon cancer, elevated cholesterol levels, and heart disease, this information is allowing saviors like Mr. Knight to look out for what is BEST for their students. I truly applaud all of the Oak Park School Board members for putting the nutrition and health of their students above all else. In this age of special interests and politics, I'm shocked and thrilled at the same time that Oak Park Schools pulled off this incredible feat. I could simply imagine some uninformed parent at a PTA meeting, or at a large school board meeting standing up in protest claiming: "My little Johnny has Type-O blood and he therefore needs to eat red meat to get his iron and protein every day". Luckily all the parents I spoke with were extremely knowledgeable about nutrition, alkalinity, etc. and spread the word throughout the school community. By the way, that whole "Type-O blood type" argument is ridiculous. In the event that this certain blood type does require a slighter higher amount of protein or iron to function better, that does NOT mean that your body needs more red meat (loaded with uric acid, cholesterol, and in some cases antibiotics, and growth hormones). To me logic would say that if this blood type does need more protein and more iron, you can get that protein and iron from many different food sources, NOT only red meat! Anyway, thank God in the case of the Oak Park School District that common sense and logic prevailed with the leadership of Mr. Knight. Let's hope that this trend continues with other schools in the future!

3. The third example is a work in progress by a small group of students at the University of California – Berkeley. I have not been able to confirm how far along this small group of students is, but apparently there is a movement to draft a California state bill next year to better allocate the use of State resources (taxpayer money) spent on food stamps. This radical bill, if it gets any traction and gets to the halls of Sacramento makes a lot of sense for the health of Californians as well as the fiscal health of the state. California now has almost $380 billion in debt – yes that's billion with a "B"! Part of the problem is with almost 2 million people unemployed, there are well over 4 million residents on food stamps in California. This is for one (1) single state! The gist of the bill these students are considering is to put restrictions on certain foods that food stamps can buy. For example: right now in California, you can't buy beer or any kind of alcohol with food stamps. The bill would recommend restricting certain types of foods and beverages that all of us (the taxpayers) are paying for. For example: eliminating about 25 "types" of foods and beverages that are non-essential for nutrition such as sodas, high octane energy drinks, candy, and desserts. There is no current law stating that people shopping in

California can't buy any of this "junk food", but the bill would propose that people could NOT use food stamps to buy their Coca-Cola and Twizzlers. I really like the logic presented because why should taxpayers keep paying for other people's junk food when millions more California residents get Type II diabetes each year? California residents who can not afford health care then get the state to pay for their diabetes treatments and medications! I haven't been able to speak to anyone at Berkeley about this, but their bill (if it gets on the ballot and eventually gets signed into law), could have huge ramifications and spread to other states which also have massive deficits in part fueled by the rising medical costs. I wish these folks all the best in advancing this novel concept. I'm not a believer of big Government ever telling its citizens what type of food, drinks, etc. they can buy with their own money, as these should be OUR rights. However, if the taxpayers of California are spending tens of billions of dollars to help feed other people, that money should be used for nutritious food and NOT for toxic food that continues to make it's population even sicker. This is common sense!

"A healthy body is the guest-chamber of the soul; a sick, its prison."
- Francis Bacon

CHAPTER FORTY-ONE (41):
Three Success Stories of Results

If you've gotten to this point where we're about to part ways and you have ANY DOUBT that you can turn your health around, here are 3 stories to confirm that almost anybody can improve their health. I could list dozens of stories about miraculous recoveries, but I'll leave you with stories of 3 individuals who were told by traditional medical doctors that their conditions could only fixed by surgery, or could not be improved at all. Yet the outcomes of these 3 individuals PROVE that the STRATEGIES IN THIS BOOK WORK!

The first story is absolutely remarkable and if anyone reading this book has any bone disease, osteoporosis, etc. it's probably not nearly as bad as this teenage kid named Sean who developed Osteogenesis Imperfecta (OI), often referred to as "brittle bone disease". There are different types and levels of brittle bone disease, but Sean's case was so bad that if he were to cough or sneeze too hard, he would break a rib. He was for the most part relegated to a life in his wheel chair and very little movement. I've worked on TV shows with people that have brittle bone disease (including Atticus Shaffer, the 13 year old actor who plays Brick on ABC's "The Middle"). Whenever I'm working in a scene with Atticus, the production staff gives all the cast & crew a reminder to NOT touch or bump Atticus because the condition makes his bones so brittle they could easily break. Getting back to Sean, his condition got so bad that he was ordered by his medical doctors not to even exercise anymore, as movement alone could break or damage his bones or joints. His case was terminal with only a few years left for him to live. Luckily, Sean crossed paths a few years ago with Tony Robbins through a "Make-A-Wish" foundation request. After Sean's wish was granted and he attended a weekend seminar event with Tony, the two of them had lunch and a long discussion about alkalinity. Tony was convinced that acidity was the major issue behind Sean's problems and urged Sean and his family to at least talk to some of the specialists in this field. Fast forward a year later and Sean showed up at another

Tony Robbins event (he wanted to surprise Tony) and Sean had completely alkalized his system and had so much energy he jumped up out of his chair and started doing full blown push ups and sit ups on the ground! Sean was high-fiving people, where just a year earlier he was afraid to slap hands or hug anyone. Sean's recovery was an extreme case, but it clearly demonstrates how powerful alkalizing one's body is with this miracle!

The second is my story. When I was little kid (around 8 years old), I used to downhill snow ski all the time growing up and eventually started downhill slalom racing when our family went to Quebec, Canada each winter. Racing down the black diamond slopes as fast as humanly possible is not the best thing for your knees, but you don't worry about these things when you're a kid. For the next 15 years, I also got into competitive waterskiing including long distance jumping. The combination of a lot of running, snow skiing and waterski jumping messed up both of my knees so bad I had to stop jogging. I couldn't even have my knees bent in a regular chair in the same position for more than 30 minutes, and God forbid I bumped my knee on an airline seat in front of me as that caused excruciating pain. Little did I know that drinking 4 – 5 Mountain Dew soft drinks (pure acid!) every day was making matters much worse. The other problem was popping 3 – 4 Advil every day when the pain got really bad. Just like many people, I just kept putting a Band-Aid on the problem, instead of addressing the symptom. After a few years of limping around, I finally consulted with the Jewett Orthopedic Clinic in Orlando, which is one of the best groups of knee surgeons in the southeast U.S. To make a long story short, I went ahead with an operation and followed up with rehab for several months. Since both knees needed arthroscopic surgery, the doctors decided to scope the right knee first so I could still walk with crutches, and then a few months later do surgery on the left knee. The surgery was much more involved then the surgeons thought and they ended up cutting the front of my leg open so they could take my entire patella (knee cap) out to work on, but in the end it was an incredible success. Fast-forward 8 months after the surgery and the rehab, and my right knee was 100% healed. It felt amazing to have full strength back in my leg along with no pain or stiffness. The plan of then having my left knee operated on (which the surgeons said was the "ONLY OPTION" to gain normal use of my knee again) was abruptly curtailed when my insurance company denied any coverage for the surgery since they claimed I had a "pre-existing condition" with my first operation! I was totally screwed and since no other insurance company (this was before Obama Care) would let me sign up for a new policy to cover this needed surgery. I was relegated to several years of one good right knee and limping along on a bum left knee. Fast forward another ten (10) years later when I really started implementing proper alkalinity and hydration techniques as spelled out in this book. Along with stretching, moderate daily exercise, and incantations, my left knee over time is also back to 100%! I can now go running, skiing, hiking, biking, etc. anytime I want. I to this day I'm amazed that my left knee without any surgery is the same, if not better than my right knee which was the one operated on!

The third story involves Christopher Reeve (aka Superman), who as you might remember had a tragic accident when he was thrown headfirst off of his horse. Christopher sustained a cervical spinal injury that paralyzed him from the neck down. The severe impact of his 215-pound body hitting the ground completely shattered his first and second vertebrae. The crushed first and second cervical vertebrae meant that Reeve's skull and spine were not connected. His desperate situation might have made him commit suicide if his good friend Robin Williams (who played Dr. "Patch Adams" in that popular film) hadn't stopped by several times in the hospital and introduced Christopher to laughter therapy. Reeve had occupational therapy and physical therapy in rehab including the use of electrodes to stimulate his muscles since he couldn't move anything below his neck. Since Reeve was relegated to this condition, this became a personal fight for him. Reeve was elected Chairman of the American Paralysis Association and later co-founded the Reeve-Irvine Research Center, now one of the leading spinal cord research centers in the world. The rule of thumb for any possible nerve regeneration from an accident like this, is there would have to be some muscle movement or feeling within 6 months after the accident. If after 2 years, there was no sign of nerve regeneration, it was thought by even the most optimistic neurologists for any recovery to be physically impossible. Reeve kept his body as physically strong as possible because he believed that the nervous system could be regenerated through intense physical therapy despite what all the doctors told him. Reeve gave daily commands (incantations) to his fingers to "move" and he visualized that one day he would regain movement of his fingers and toes. One day (five years after his accident) Christopher actually regained some motor function including movement in his fingers and toes, could raise his right arm, and was able to sense hot and cold temperatures on his body! Upon revealing this miracle the medical world had never witnessed before Reeve commented on his doctor, John McDonald's reaction: "I don't think Dr. McDonald would have been more surprised if I had just walked on water!". Sadly Reeve died a few years later from an antibiotic drug that was administered to him, but he was the true model of a "Superman" until the very end.

I would love to hear about your success story. Just go back and re-read any section of the book as needed or advance to the Appendix where you can find the step by step process of how to start the 7-Day "Alkalize & Energize" cleanse including a FAQ page we've developed after working with over 50 people this far. If you have no support system to help you get started, Nemours Marketing now offers consultation & coaching (over the phone, Skype, or i-Chat) to help walk you though the first 7 days, and the next month or two if you want to continue for a modest fee. Our contact information is listed at the end of this book, so please call or e-mail if you'd like help regaining your perfect health! If you don't choose us, and you feel you need a coach (even for just a short time), make SURE you choose a doctor, a nutritionist, a health expert, or a trainer who is in EXCELLENT HEALTH. It disturbs me when I see an overweight doctor telling their patients to go on a special diet, or a flabby gym trainer telling his or her clients how to get in perfect shape. This should be common sense, but just a reminder that if you want a successful outcome, work with someone who has already gotten the RESULTS you want.

"In a disordered mind, as in a disordered body, soundness of health is impossible."
- Cicero

CHAPTER FORTY-TWO (42):
You Decide Where to Go From Here...

Thank you for taking the time to read this new book and I applaud you for taking a major step towards reclaiming your health. These 5 topics and tools WILL help you live a longer, healthier, & more energetic life. At this point, it's up to YOU to decide where to go from here. There are two ways you can move forward:

1) Continue to take prescription drugs, consult with your doctor about surgical options, and look into the new fads such as new lap-band (financing now available for just $79 per month), liposuction, fat freezing, gastric bypass surgery, etc.

2) Make a bold decision right now to do the 7-Day "Alkalize & Energize" cleanse to start regaining your health! After the 7 days, you can make the conscious effort to eat an 80% alkaline diet, oxygenate your system, start exercising (even if using your NET time), and develop a faith that you can "regain great health"!

A third choice (although I did not list it as an option), and hope you do NOT fall into this trap, is for you to close the book right now and say to yourself: "nice book, I learned a few things", but then fail to follow through and take action! This is the road often traveled where people fall into mediocrity. You justify why you can't exercise today, and tell yourself that you'll start "tomorrow". You're at a cocktail party with some old friends and after a few servings of salami, cheese, and crackers you have some chocolate truffles and then one last after dinner drink while smoking a cigar to wind down for the evening. Once again, you tell yourself that you'll eat better tomorrow or someday soon. The problem is that "someday soon" often leads you down the river of life to "nowhere". The solution is to right NOW do one of two things. First, tell your spouse, a family member, or a really good friend (someone you trust will support you) that you are doing the 7-Day cleanse and you've decided you're going to get healthy NOW! If you can't tell that person right now, make a phone call to that person so you make the commitment and you have leverage. I was working on a TV show with my friend Bruce Ellington while he was eating a pastry and to be honest he was not looking his best. But despite his skepticism about the program, he got HONEST with himself (about his sweet tooth, his extra weight, his lack of energy, etc.) and he made the phone call right then and there to his wife Jill that he was going to start the 7-Day "Alkalize & Energize" cleanse the very next day. Thank you Jill for supporting your husband and helping get him back on track to amazing health! The second option, if you can't call someone at this very moment, is to take out a notepad or your day planner, and write down a list of 5 health goals you want to achieve in the next 30 days. As proven many times in this book, you will get results fairly quickly (some in the first 7 days and substantial results in about 30 days). How much weight do you want to lose? What healthy food choices are you going to make, and what junk foods are you going to eliminate or at least scale back? What kind of exercise are you going to start tomorrow? What NET activity will you start doing daily without requiring any extra more time in your busy schedule? If you're like my older brother, he just implemented his new routine of walking up or down 10 flights of stairs every time he comes and goes from his office building. He feels great and it often doesn't take any extra time when he considers the time he used to wait for just a few stops the elevator would make. As Nike's famous slogan reads around the world: "JUST DO IT!".

Which ever steps you take right now (as soon as you finish this book), for long term success, make sure you have a support system (a spouse, family member, good friend, etc.) who will support your efforts. Make an effort to start cleaning all the junk food out of your house. Some of the people we've worked with now refer to packaged or processed foods as "poison" and some even discarded those foods in a celebration ceremony on their way to perfect health.

Also, don't forget to start each day off with empowering questions and incantations. As you learned throughout Section V, you can change your emotional (and physical) state first thing in the morning to set the tone for a great day, a great week, and a great month, which will set you up for a great life! When you first start this process if you need to write a cue card to place by your bedside, that's OK, these empowering morning questions are probably a new concept for you, but here are a few sample questions you can start with:

1) How am I lucky enough in this economy to still have a job?

2) Why am I still alive when my roommate (cousin, brother, etc.) died of cancer?

3) How did I get fortunate enough to have family (or great friends) who love me?

4) How lucky am I to live in the United States (one of the most prosperous nations in the world), while millions of less fortunate people live in impoverished nations with severe food shortages and limited drinkable water?

5) How was I chosen at this point in time to sleep last night on a bed, with a roof over my head, and have access to clean water to shower or bathe in, have electricity for air conditioning, and have a refrigerator right in my house filled with food?

These are just a few sample questions you can ask every day. Also make sure you set the bar low at first, so you don't make it too difficult for yourself to feel grateful each day. If you are one of the brave veterans coming back from Iraq with both of your legs amputated, maybe you could ask the question: "How was I lucky enough to keep both of my arms?" I don't want to belittle how terrible a tragedy it must be to have lost both your legs, but isn't better to ask an empowering question or compare yourself to Tisha Shelton who was born a congenital amputee with no arms and no legs. I met Tisha on the set of the Jeff Probst show a few months ago and she was such an inspiration utilizing daily empowering questions she asks herself. She focuses on what she HAS vs. what she doesn't have.

All of the rituals in this book (including eating healthy alkaline foods, oxygenating your body, asking empowering questions, and implementing NET exercise, etc.) can last a lifetime once you start doing them. Congratulations to you in advance for regaining your perfect health! I look forward from hearing from you about YOUR own success story...

⇔ SUBSTITUTE: The next time you have any doubts about anything including your body, your diet, etc. pause for a moment. Don't compare your body or your health to anyone else's, but instead think about the small steps you ARE taking in terms of your diet, exercise, thoughts, etc. and have absolute faith that you ARE making progress in the right direction every single day!

Appendix:

7- Day "Alkalize & Energize"
Cleanse notes:

Day 1 - 7:
(Almost all people do 7 days. You can extend to 10 days if you wish)

1 - 2 (16 oz.) large glasses of alkaline, filtered water with lemon slices 1st thing in the morning.

1 (16 oz.) large glass of fresh cucumber, spinach, carrot, broccoli, juice for breakfast*

8 - 10 large glasses (or bottles) of alkaline, filtered water with lemon throughout the day.

1 (16 oz.) large glass of fresh cucumber, spinach, carrot, broccoli, juice for lunch if hungry.

2 - 3 "Green" drinks during the day. Mix 2 teaspoons or 1 small scoop of powdered greens in your water bottle.*

1 small cup of raw, unsalted, all natural almonds (chewed completely before swallowing). This is a great snack w-protein.

1 -2 Cups of "Green" Tea (with lemon for flavor, but NO sugar, honey, Agave, or sweeteners of any kind).

1 (16 oz.) glass of celery, green squash, carrot, green pepper juice for dinner.

ADDITIONAL NOTES:
Do NOT eat any fruits or drink any fruit juice for 7 days – they have sugar (& any trace amount of sugar is acidic)!

You can mix different vegetables each day if you want. Try squash, zucchini, green beans, kale, sprouts, etc.

Stay away from frozen, cooked, or processed vegetables as they have less nutritional value & can be acidic.

Make sure you DON'T drink any store bought canned vegetable juice. V-8 and other brands are loaded with potassium chloride, sugar, magnesium, ascorbic acid, citric acid, added salt & lots of preservatives.

On Day 5, start drinking 2 – 3 glasses of water mixed with Metamucil (w- Psyllium husks) each day.

Your system should be completely cleaned out & detoxified by day 7.

*Fruit exception: you may use a ¼ apple slice if needed in your vegetable juice for the first 2 – 3 days, if the taste is too bitter.

*Fruit juice exception: you may add 1 – 2 oz. of apple juice into "Green" powdered drink the first 2 – 3 days, if the taste is too bitter.

Additional Quotes from Medical Experts:

"Up to 90% of diseases are due to improper functioning of the colon.... Of the 22,000 operations that I have performed, I have never found a single normal colon."

- Dr. John Harvey Kellogg

"Every physician should realize that the intestinal toxemia (poisons) are the most important primary and contributing causes of many disorders and diseases of the human body."

- Gastroenterologist, Dr. Anthony Bassler

"More than 65 different health challenges are caused by a toxic colon."

- The Royal Society of Medicine of Great Britain

"3.6 Years can be added to your life by cutting most meat out of your diet."

- American Journal of Clinical Nutrition

"The heavy mucus coating in the colon thickens and becomes a host of putrefaction. The blood capillaries to the colon begin to pick up the toxins, poisons and noxious debris as it seeps through the bowel wall. All tissues and organs of the body are now taking on toxic substances. Here is the beginning of true autointoxication on a physiological level. ... Autointoxication is self-poisoning, or slow suicide. Through detoxification, proper nutrition, and administration of supplements, the body can heal itself and maintain optimum health function."

- Nobel Prize Nominee, Dr. Bernard Jensen DC, ND, Ph.D

7-Day "Alkalize & Energize" (Cleanse)
Common Mistakes:

Common Mistake:	Typical Example(s):	Explanation:
1a. "Cheating"	Eating a banana or having 1 glass of wine (these are usually influenced by friends or family who are unhealthy themselves).	Even a small amount of sugar (in fruit or alcohol) will not allow your body to fully alkalize.
1b. Lying to yourself	Telling yourself that 1 piece of candy won't matter and you can make it up in the morning.	NA
2. Starvation mode	Juicing only once a day.	If you don't get enough calories, your body will NOT drop weight, but instead retain that fat as a defense mechanism called "starvation mode".
3. Allowing an old habit to interfere	Smoking	Smoking anything (legal or not) is not good for you & ANY smoke you put into your moth or lungs is acidic.
4. Not "alkalizing" enough.	In addition to juicing, you should be drinking at least 2 – 3 "Green" Drinks each day (either powdered "Green" drink or wheat grass).	It takes 4 parts alkalinity to counter 1 part acidity. During the 7-day cleanse, you need to super-alkalize your system to allow your boy to start losing weight.
5. Too much extreme physical exercise!	Sneaking into the gym one day to lift weights, doing wind sprints, or a long endurance run.	Almost nobody believes or understands this, but trust us this is TRUE. Any extreme exercise will create lactic acid in your system and then you are back to square

		one.
6a. Not getting enough exercise.	Besides walking up the stairs in their house or walking down the hallway at work, most people do NOT get real daily exercise anymore.	The key to start removing acids and toxins from your body is muscle movement and aerobic exercise. Walking several miles, doing a gentle 30 – 45 minute hike, going on a long bicycle ride, doing a yoga class, etc. will.
6b. Taking in more calories than you are burning.	Taking in 2,000 calories each day and only burning 1,900.	Common sense – if you are not exercising enough to burn off the calories you are intaking each day, these excess calories will be stored as fat. This is normally how people gain weight in the 1st place!
7. Juicing late at night or right before you go to bed.	NA	Common sense would dictate NOT to give your body lots of alkaline nutrition when trying to wind down & go to sleep.
8. Irregular sleep pattern	Walking up & going to bed at different times every day.	A regular sleep pattern will allow your body cells to rest & recover each day. Not getting enough sleep can make your body acidic.
9. Negative thoughts or stress.	This could even be ANY negative "vocabulary" that you use when speaking such as: "I am so stupid".	Just because you did 1 stupid thing, does not mean you are stupid!
10. Continuing to take vitamins, supplements, etc.	Do not take any supplements of vitamins unless your doctor says you must.	Vitamins and other supplements often have sugar, and other chemicals added to them. These 7 days you want to clean all of that out of your system!

Frequently Asked Questions (FAQ):

Q: What is the 7-Day "Alkalize & Energize" Cleanse Program?

A: This is 7-Day Liquid Cleanse that will "Alkalize & Energize" your body. We do not want to underestimate how much better you feel in just 7 days, but for any skeptics, we will provide "before" & "after" photos of both authors who have done this many times before. The 50+ other people who have also done this cleanse as well all had dramatic results & took photos they kept for themselves. The U.S. leads all developed countries with over 66% of the population overweight & 30% of the population morbidly obese! If you are part of these statistics, this program will help.

Q: What is the Best Time to Get Started?

A: Right Now! Most people in the U.S. have built up toxins & poisons in their body through added chemicals, 3rd generation pesticides, antibiotics, steroids, super growth hormones, excess sugars, additives & preservatives that were not in our foods just 25 years ago. The only time we do NOT recommend to start this would be over the Holidays being surrounded by all the sweets, sugar treats, excessive food, coffee & alcohol.

Q: What do I Need to Get Started?

A:

1. A Vegetable Juicer – you can borrow one, or else you can find one for $60 - $80 at Wal-Mart or about $25 on Craig's List or e-Bay will get you a nice used one.

2. "Green" Powdered Drink – you can buy from a health food store, Vitamin Shoppe, etc. A medium size container will last you a few months & should cost between $15 - $25. It is important to make sure this powder is only "Greens" with NO added sugar, corn syrup, fructose, or any additives. Also do NOT buy any Green drink that has any berries or fruit added.

3. Alkaline Water – if you're not purchasing alkaline water or have a Kangen™ type of water system, we recommend you at least use a filtration system that mounts on your

kitchen faucet, or an inexpensive Britta™ type of water pitcher-filter system. You should add lemon slices to your glass or pitcher, which will alkalize the water. Also add 1 ice cube to each glass of alkaline water when you drink. The ice cube will slowly change from a solid state to a liquid state, giving you a slight bit of energy.

4. Fresh Vegetables you can find in your local farmer's market or grocery store. Buy organic when possible. If you cannot afford organic, make sure you carefully wash all vegetables before juicing.

5. Fresh Lemons to add to your water. Do NOT add store bought lemon juice!

6. Green Tea - especially if you are a coffee drinker & feel you need a little caffeine. You may substitute "green" tea for coffee this week. Make sure the tea you get is all natural with has no added sugars or flavorings.

7. Psyllium Husk (most common brand is Metamucil). A small container of powdered Psyllium Husk is more than enough as you are only taking this the last 2 days of your cleanse.

8. Raw Almonds – a great alkaline protein snack for this week. Get a small bag or can of almonds & make sure there are raw & NOT roasted or salted & there is no sugar or added flavors.

Q: Will I Get Hungry at all or Have Food Cravings?
A: You might have some minor cravings the 1st or 2nd day if you have Yeast & Candida in your system. The candida feed on sugars, processed foods and acids, which you will be eliminating. If you do the program exactly as we recommend & drink LOTS of water and powdered "Green" drink in between your meals, you should not feel any hunger after the 2nd day. Part of the hunger is "psychological" with not eating solid foods and missing the act of eating. If you should feel a little hungry, drink a tall glass or bottle of water, or another bottle of Green drink. It is critical to have a water and/or "Green" drink in front of you at ALL times. This week you will be super-hydrating your system.

Q: How I Can Get Enough Nutrition From one 16 – 20 oz. Glass of Juice compared to the Large Portions of Food I 'm Used to Eating?

A: Since the vegetable juice you drink is all-natural and loaded with natural nutrition, vitamins, proteins, & minerals your body can easily digest & quickly assimilate, this will provide as much (if not more energy) than a huge meal that your body can not fully utilize. This is common sense.

Q: What if I Have a Business Lunch or a Planned Outing with Food?

A: There is nothing wrong with ordering a glass of lemon water or an Green tea with lemon and explain you are not hungry. If it is too awkward at a big business meeting to not eat anything, you may have a bowl of split pea soup or a green salad with NO dressing. For dressing you can add some lemon juice and a dash of ground black pepper. Make sure the salad has no fruits in it (no raisins, cranberries, apples, etc. as these fruits contain lots of sugar). If you feel compelled to eat a salad one day for a business lunch, etc. you do NOT need to "fall off the wagon" and stop your cleanse! Just make sure you chew the lettuce, cucumbers, broccoli, etc. very slowly & completely before you swallow. As you continue chewing, the more pepsin & renin (digestive enzymes) will be released to help break the salad down closer towards a liquid state.

Q: What Are the Main Rules (and any Foods to Avoid) for these 7 Days?

A: You're going to eat (actually drink) all ALKALINE foods. Mostly green vegetables, sprouts, etc. and powdered Green drink that you mix with water. You must avoid all acidic foods (processed refined foods, meats, dairy, fruits, bread, pasta, sugars, etc.) to cleanse & detox your system.

Q: Why Can't I Eat Fruit... I Heard Fruit was a Healthy Food?

A: Fruits are healthy foods, but most fruits are loaded with sugar. To properly "alkalize" you do not want to consume any fruits or fruit juices (and all these sugars) for the 1st 7 days while you're on this cleanse. You may be tempted to eat one banana or an avocado, but you must NOT eat any fruit for these 7 days.

Q: Will I Really Feel That Much Better?

A: Yes! We've asked all the other people who have done this program to describe in a journal how they feel after the 5th or 6th day. Here is how some of our friends & family have described their health and energy after just a few days: "energized, alive, super-charged, new vitality, vigor, stamina, bouncing off the walls, excited, happy, renewed, rejuvenated, happy, healthy, like the fountain of youth!"

Q: I'm on Prescription Drugs & Take Several "Over the Counter" Medications. Should I Stop Taking Them?

A: You are not alone. 48% of all Americans now take prescription drugs on a regular basis and almost 90% of people over the age of age of 70 take some kind of prescription drugs! Most of this is due to an acidic diet & lack of exercise. You should NOT change your regiment of prescriptions unless you talk to your doctor. Many people who have done this program have gotten off most of their prescriptions & medications. Some over time have completely stopped taking all their medications! Remember that it may take several weeks or months to get off your medications, & you should always consult with your doctor, as your body gets more alkaline & back towards a state of perfect health.

Q: Can I Stop Taking Vitamins and Store Bought Supplements?

A: Unless your doctor has specifically told you to take certain vitamins or supplements, you should not take these during the 7-day cleanse. The natural vitamins, minerals, and overall nutrition you'll get from the vegetable juice & green drink will be more than what your body needs. In reality, in many cases the store bought vitamins & supplements from pharmaceutical companies simply ends up being expensive urine.

Q: Why Should I Have a Journal or Make Notes?

A: In addition to taking a photo & weighing yourself before you start & after Day 7 (these "before" & "after" photos will be show some of your physical results), you'll want to write down a few notes each day on how you feel & what signals your body is telling you. We had one gentleman who had a large cut that scabbed up & while on the cleanse, it completely healed in just 3 days. This man was so acidic before the cleanse, it used to take him 2 – 3 weeks for a cut to completely heal!

Q: What Should I Do After the 1st 7 Days?

A: Please call us & we can discuss which route you want to go. We've had some friends continue juicing for many months who have lost 60, even 100lbs!, but most importantly they feel better & healthier every single day. Other people prefer getting back to a solid-food diet & we can walk you through a plan where you can go back to a regular food diet, that 80% alkaline which will help you maintain the great health you should be feeling after just 7 days. The choice is yours.

Q: Why Do I Lose So Much Weight so Quickly?

A: Most people with a "western" diet (especially in the U.S.) are eating lots of processed & refined foods loaded with sugars & meats, which are very acidic. To check your acidity before your cleanse, you can either have a blood test done, or buy a simple pH strip test (sold at your local pharmacy) to test your ph level before you start. The main reason people in this country are obese (and there are millions of morbidly obese people in the U.S. today) is that their body's natural defense against extra acid is to store lots of fat. This extra fat protects your body including all the vital organs. In just a few days, when your body starts becoming more & more alkaline, you will start shedding pounds even without a lot of exercise. Every single person who has done this program has lost 1 – 4 lbs. each day!

Q: Why Can't I Do a Lot of Physical Exercise?

A: We recommend NOT lifting heavy weights, doing wind sprints, or super long runs as these activities will produce lactic acid in your system. Daily exercise such as walking, biking, hiking, or even moderate jogging are fine & recommended. Any kind of yoga, stretching or exercise where you doing deep diaphragmatic breathing is excellent as these breathing exercises will activate your lymphatic system to help clean out the toxins in your body. Sitting in a steam room or a sauna for a limited time is also fine as this will help toxins escape your body.

Q: At Certain Times During the Day I Feel Tired... Is this Normal?

A: Most likely you're not drinking enough Green Drink (which is pure alkaline energy). We've also noticed (with time capture cameras) people sitting motionless at their computers for 3 - 4 hours at a time. If your only body part moving is your mouse finger, it's no surprise you will feel tired! Make a point of standing up every 30 minutes & taking a quick break every hour or two. This is common sense! A great tip to make sure you do this is to set the timer on your cell phone for 90 minutes or write your break time on a post-it note by your computer screen. To keep your energy level up, you NEED to get up at least every 90 minutes to get more water, take a bathroom break, etc. On Day or 6 or 7 (when the Metamucil is working through your colon), you may feel a little tired until you discharge. Some people in our studies on Day 7 have lost 5 – 10lbs! This is painless, and you should feel amazing after that bulk of toxins & fecal matter has completely passed.

Q: Are You Sponsored by Any Company(s) or Products?

A: No. Both authors of this book have lost close relatives & friends the past few years to cancer & disease. We're sharing this information to help others re-gain the excellent health everyone deserves. Although heart disease, arthritis, high cholesterol, obesity, acid reflux, muscle & joint pains are "common" for people in the U.S., this was not "normal" 50 years ago. One of the authors worked for Medco (one of the largest prescription drug fulfillment companies in the U.S.) for 8 years & will tell you from personal experience the amount of prescription drugs that even young people are now taking (people in their 20s in 30s) has increasing dramatically the last 2 years. The U.S. Government & private companies burdened with these expensive health care costs are finally realizing that a better solution to start getting their employees healthier is though better diet & exercise.

Q: I've Been Doing the Cleanse for 3 Days and Haven't Lost Any Weight?

A: See the attached table, but there are four (4) main reasons:

    1...You are cheating with a piece of fruit or a glass of fruit juice. Even a few raisins or cranberries have a lot of sugar in them. You can NOT have any sugar for these 7 days, as excess sugar will convert to acid.

    2. You are not having 3 meals (or drinks) per day. If you try and "cheat" and don't take nutritional calories in every 5 – 6 hours, your body will go into "starvation" mode and will not release any of it's fat. This is why most low calorie or depriving diets don't work.

    3. You're drinking too much vegetable juice. If you are drinking large amounts of juice at one time (20 – 25 ounces is too much), not only will you have expensive urine, but your body may store some of this excess nutrition in the form of fat.

    4. You worked out too hard! Both authors made this mistake by lifting heavy weights during a cleanse. Neither lost any weight those days, and in fact Scott gained 1.4 lbs. in one day due to the fact that an intense workout like sprinting or lifting weights creates lots of "lactic acid" in your body. That lactic acid in turn signals your body to keep storing fat to protect your vital organs from this new acid in your system.

Q: Any last Minute Tips?

A: Yes. Do not put your water pitcher in the refrigerator. You'll be drinking so much water each day (2 – 4 liters) & you don't want to chill your core body too much. It's better to drink room temperature water. However, we do recommend putting 1 small ice cube into the water you drink. This won't chill the water that much but as the cube transforms from a "solid" state to a "liquid" state of energy, it will help energize you! Also, you should stop drinking water at least 1 hour before you go to bed. Drinking an extra 2 – 3 large glasses of water right before going to sleep may cause you to use the rest room during the night. Also if you notice the 3rd or 4th day your feet smell, or you have a little body odor, that is natural. That smell is the toxins (which have built up in your body over many years) finally escaping!

Q: How Do I Continue After the Cleanse?

A: If you stop the cleanse after 7 days, 10 days, or 30 days, you then want to transition to a healthy lifestyle diet which is sustainable LONG-TERM. Simply ensure that 80 – 90% of your diet (all foods, beverages, snacks, etc.) is alkaline. The easiest way is to make sure that most of your diet is made up of vegetables and a limited amount of fruits. There are several charts including a great one by Dr. Theodore Baroody in his book Alkalize or Die, but here is a very comprehensive chart:
www.acidalkalinediet.com/Alkaline-Foods-Chart.htm. As long as MOST of your diet is alkaline and healthy, you should still be able to have that slice of birthday cake, pumpkin pie, or chocolate chip cookie now and then on special occasions.

Q: Can You Share Some Recipes or Examples of What You Eat After the Cleanse?

A: We strongly suggest you invest in a healthy (alkaline) cookbook or get one from your local library. Instead of turning this into a full-blown recipe book, we simply wanted to educate you and point you in the right direction. With that said, here is a sample of what Scott & Ronald (contributing author) eat on a regular basis:

Breakfast (an hour or so after several glasses of alkaline water):
Vegetable-Fruit Smoothie. In a blender add 1 cup of apple juice, 1 banana, ½ large cucumber, 1 small green pepper, 1 tablespoon of vanilla yogurt, 1 tablespoon of organic Tofu, 1 teaspoon of organic Agave sweetener, 2 ice cubes. Fill the top of the blender with filtered water depending on how many people the drink is serving.

Lunch:
Large salad with lots of greens and alkaline vegetables. You can sprinkle in a small handful of cranberries, raisins, and blueberries if desired. For dressing only use a tiny amount of extra virgin olive oil & balsamic vinegar and then add lots of fresh squeezed lemon juice on top as well for some zest.

A great soup combo to go with this salad is split-pea soup with which you can add in minced celery, mushrooms, or spinach for extra protein.

For a drink, have a nice glass of **Green Tea** sweetened with lemon or a little Agave.

Dinner:
Black Bean Taco Soup. 1 can of natural black beans (no sugar or sodium added). Slice up onions, mushrooms, Roma tomatoes, 1 avocado and simmer. Add soup over organic, unsalted taco chips. Add a dash of black pepper if desired and sprinkle basil and parsley flakes on top and serve warm.

For a drink try a combination $1/3^{rd}$ apple juice and $1/3^{rd}$ cranberry-pomegranate juice with the top $1/3^{rd}$ of the glass topped off with filtered water. The water will slightly dilute the high sugar content found in the juices.

Early evening snack:
1 glass of **red wine** with **some green snap-peas,** or you can try a small bowl piece of **fresh, ripe fruit**.

⇔SUBSTITUTE: The next time you're tempted to skip your daily walk, or drink a 64 oz. big Gulp soda, break the pattern by calling a friend (or your coach) for support. One small step such as talking to a positive friend for 5 minutes can break your negative pattern and get you back on track!

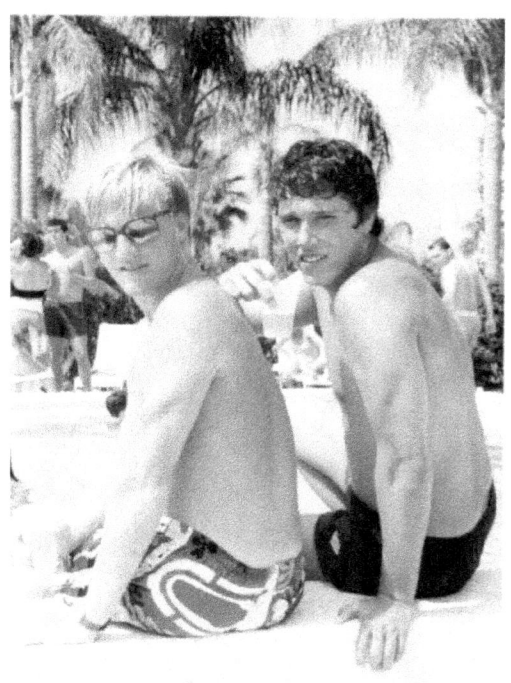

PHI DELTA THETA
With fraternity brother & college roommate (John Clark)
poolside at a spring weekend event. RIP my friend.

General Info:
Nemours Marketing, Inc.
info@nemoursmarketing.com
www.nemoursmarketing.com
Tel: (310) 855 - 9355
Fax: (360) 656 - 7268

Live Coaching Services:
Nemours Marketing, Inc.
ScottduP@juno.com
www.nemoursmarketing.com
Tel: (407) 738 - 1608
Fax: (360) 656 – 7268

Reference Notes:

F-1 Stand Up 2 Cancer (SU2C.com) June, 2012.

F-2 "Too Fat to Fight" www.dailymail.co.uk , By Larissa Brown, December 11, 2012

1-1 "USA is Fattest of 33 Countries" article by Nanci Hellmich, USA Today, September 23, 2010.

1-2 "The Heart Disease Trifecta". Los Angeles Times article by Thomas H. Maugh II, April 26, 2010.

1-3 "Diabetes May Affect 1 in 3 by 2050." USA Today article by Mary Brophy Marcus. October 22, 2010.

1-4 "Prescription Drugs Doubled in Less Than a Decade". USA Today Article by Robert Preidt. September 4, 2010.

1-5. Food is Your Best Medicine Henry G. Bieler, M.D. Published 1966 Random House, Inc. p. 255

1-6. "Ohio Puts 200-pound Third-Grader in Foster Care." ABC News report November 28, 2011 ABC News

3-1 "Forks Over Knives", 2011 Monica Beach Productions

3-2 "Forks Over Knives", 2011 Monica Beach Productions

3-3 "Forks Over Knives", 2011 Monica Beach Productions

3-4 "Genetic Roulette: The Gable of Our Lives", 2012 The Institute for Responsible Technology

3-5 "Genetic Roulette: The Gable of Our Lives", 2012 The Institute for Responsible Technology

3-6 "GMO Food Allergies" www.HubPages.com blog 11-20-12 by MagicStarER

3-7 "American Per-Capita Sugar Consumption Hits 100 Pounds Per Year". by Henry Blodget, www.Businessinsider.com. February 19th, 2012.

3-8. "Youth Diabetes, Pre-diabetes Rates Soar". USA Today article by Nanci Hellmich, May 20, 2012.

4-1 "The Alkalarian Approach to Optimal Health" by Dr. Robert and Shelley Young from www.pHMiracleLiving.com .

6-1 "Weight Issues" Time Magazine, page 11. July 9, 2012.

6-2 The pH Miracle: Balance Your Diet, Reclaim Your Health
Robert O. Young, PhD. and Shelley Redford Young, June, 2008

7-1 Merriam-Webster dictionary (www.Merriam-Webster.com)

7-2 p. 55 Toxemia Explained – The True Interpretation of the Cause of Disease J. H. Tilden, M. D., Published 1935 J.H. Tilden

9-1 Fuel – The Energy You Need to Succeed. Wes Beavis, Powerborn, 2009.

10-1 WebMD Health News, "The 10 Most Prescribed Drugs". April 20th, 2011. by Daniel J. DeNoon, Reviewed by Laura J. Martin, MD

11-1 "Can We Live Forever?" Television program by

Nova Science Now, 2011.

13 –1 It's My Life! I Can Change If I Want To, Richard D. Walker p.106, 2000

13-2 www.EstelletobyGoldstein.com, "About" p. 1. © 2012.

13-3 "Youth Diabetes, Pre-diabetes Rates Soar". USA Today article by Nanci Hellmich, May 20, 2012.

13-4 "Study: Half of U.S. Adults Will be Obese by 2030". HealthDay article by Toby Talbot, August 28, 2011.

15-1 www.NaturalCleansingTechniques.com Dr. Morris F. Keller

16-1 www.BeWellBuzz.com "Exposed: The Business Of Cancer" Podcast with Ty Bollinger, May 17th, 2012.

18-1 "Lymphatic System Drainage Part 1" YouTube video posted by www.BalancedHealthToday.com.

24- 1 Energistics, by Phyllis Paulette 1987 Paperjacks p.81

24- 2 The Food Revolution, by John Robbins 2001 Conari press p.236

24- 3 The Food Revolution, by John Robbins 2001 Conari press p.14

25-1 "Obesity fight needs ambitious campaign, health leaders say" by Judith Graham, Kaiser Health News, May 5, 2012.

25-2 "Ohio puts 200-pound third-grader in foster care" ABC News, November 28, 2011

25-3 "Obese teen had to be cut from home in U.K." by Anthony Stone Associated Press, May 25, 2012

27-1 **"America's Waistline is Growing – Again".** Time Magazine p. 14 August 27, 2012.

27-2 "Most Americans don't get daily exercise, survey finds". by Robert Preidt, Health Day. October 3, 2010.

29-1 www.MedScape.com "The Price of False Beliefs - Unrealistic Expectations as a Contributor to the Health Care Crisis". by Steven H. Woolf, MD, Nov 28, 2012

29-2 "Health Insurance Costs Rising Sharply This Year, Study Shows" by Reed Abelson, The New York Times, September 27, 2011

32-1 "Retiring at 55 Increases Death Risk in New Study", www.SeniorJournal.com, October 21, 2005.

33-1 "Insomnia Statistics", www.Better-Sleep-Better-Life.com

34-1 "Lawyers and Settlements" January, 2007

34-2 Centers for Disease Control and Prevention, NCHS Data Brief Number 76, October 2011

36-1 Positive Energy, Judith Orloff, M.D. 2004, Harmony Books

37-1 **The Auschwitz Volunteer: Beyond Bravery** – by Captain Witold Pilecki
Published by Aquila Polonica, 2012

38-1 www.naturalhormoneclinic.com Dr. Robert E. Battmer, November 21, 2012

38-2 <u>Positive Energy</u>, Judith Orloff, M.D., Harmony Books, 2004

"Sickness is the vengeance of nature
for the violation of her laws."
- Charles Simmons

Photo Credits:

<u>All photos are property of </u>Scott duPont, Inc. or Nemours Marketing, Inc. unless listed otherwise underneath photograph.

<u>Cover photo</u> courtesy of the TV show "Dr. G. Medical Examiner" and the Discovery Health Channel.

"Cancer grows and spreads in anaerobic
and acidic conditions.
Cancer is almost never found in oxygenated,
alkaline environments.
The National Cancer Institute was conceived in 1937,
but with our acidic diets
cancer rates in the U.S. continue to climb!"
- Tony Robbins

Bibliography
(Recommended Reading):

The 30-Day Diabetes Miracle Cookbook, Bonnie House & Dianna Flemming, PhD, LDN, Perigee © 2008

Alkalize or Die, Dr. Theodore A. Baroody, Holographic Health Press ©1991

Alzheimers Disease: What if There Was a Cure?, Mary T. Neport, M.D. Basic Health Publications © 2011

The Auschwitz Volunteer: Beyond Bravery, Captain Witold Pilecki, Aquila Polonica © 2012

Biomarkers – The 10 Keys to Prolonging Vitality, William Evans, M.D., Simon & Schuster © 1991

Breast Cancer – Beyond Convention, Mary Tagliferri, M.D. Atria Books © 2002

Cancer – Step Outside the Box Ty Bollinger © 2006

Childhood Cancer Survivors, Nancy Keene, O'Reilly © 2000

The Complete Encyclopedia of Natural Healing, Gary Null PhD. © 2005

Creating Health, Deepak Choprah, M.D., Houghton Mifflin © 1991

Curing Fatigue, David S. Bell, M.D. St. Martin's Press ©1993

Energistics, Phyllis Paulette, Paperjacks © 1987

Fit for Life, Harvey and Marilyn Diamond, Warner Books ©1987

Food is Your Best Medicine, Henry G. Bieler, M.D., Random House, Inc. © 1966

The Food Revolution, by John Robbins, Conari Press © 2001

Forever Young, Dr. Nicholas Perricone, Atria Books © 2010

Fuel – The Energy You Need to Succeed, Wes Beavis, Powerborn © 2009.

The Gerson Therapy, Charlotte Gerson and Morton Walker, Kensington Publishing © 2001

Healing Foods, Patricia Hausman, Dell ©1989

Healing the Gerson Way, Charlotte Gerson and Beata Bishop, Totality Books © 2009.

It's My Life! I Can Change If I Want To, Richard D. Walker © 2011

Jamie's Food Revolution: Rediscover How to Cook Simple, Delicious, Affordable Meals, Jamie Oliver © 2011

May All Be Fed, John Robbins, Morrow © 1992

Natural Cures "They" Don't Want You To Know About, Kevin Trudeau © 2006

The New Fit or Fat, Covert Bailey, Houghton Miiflin Company © 1991

The Omnivore's Dilemma, Michael Pollan. © 2007

Our Toxic World, Doris J. Rapp, M.D., Environmental Medical Research Foundation © 2004

The pH Miracle: Balance Your Diet, Reclaim Your Health Robert O. Young, PhD. and Shelley Redford Young. © 2008

Positive Energy, Judith Orloff, M.D., Harmony Books © 2004

Real Age, Michael F. Roizen, M.D., Cliff Street Books © 2000

The Relation of Alimentation and Disease, Dr. James R. Salisbury © 1888

Reversing Fibromyalgia, Dr. Joe M. Elrod, Woodland Publishing © 2002

Self Test Nutrition Guide, Dr. Cass Igram, Knowledge House © 1994

Stand Tall: Every Woman's Guide to Preventing Osteoporosis, Morris Notelovitz, Bantam Dell Publishing Group © 1985

Surgery and Its Alternatives, Sandra McLanahan, M.D., Twin Stream Books © 2002

Tarascon Pocket Pharmacopedia, Jones & Bartlett © 2012

The Total Cancer Wellness Guide, Kim Thiboldeaux, BenBella Books © 2007

Toxemia Explained – The True Interpretation of the Cause of Disease J. H. Tilden, M. D., © 1935
The Ultimate Healing System: The Illustrated Guide to Muscle Testing & Nutrition, Gary Null PhD. © 1998
A Week in the Zone, Barry Sears, Ph.D. Harper Paperbacks © 2000

Walking with the Power, Dexter Clay, Black Eye World Publishing © 2004

Your Body's Many Cries for Water, F. Batmanghelidj, M.D., Global Health Solutions © 1997

"Take care of your body.
It's the only place you have to live."
- Jim Rohn

In Loving Memory Of...

George M. Bapis

Thomas Brummett

Dr. George F. Cahill

Sarah duPont Cahill

Fritz Collister

John "Clarkey" Clark

Ronald Robert Farnham

Angelo Forgione

Dorothy Forgione

Ione "Tony" Holloway Graves

Thomas M. Green III

Thomas M. Green IV

Patsy Harris

Cindy Kramer

Christine Kyle

George L. Lee

John L. Lee, Jr.

John L. Lee

Todd Lee

Steven John Richey

Frank Shapins

Craig Soldinger

Daniel Vovak

"Health of body and mind is a great blessing,
if we can bear it."
- John Henry Cardinal Newman

100% TOTAL SATISFACTION GUARANTEE:

If for ANY reason you are not 100% satisfied with the book or DVD you purchased, just send the product back along with receipt (or proof of payment). We will gladly refund 100% of your money, no questions asked!

Nemours Marketing, Inc.
7531 Azurebrook Court
Winter Park, FL 32792
info@NemoursMarketing.com
Tel: (407) 738 - 1608

www.ingramcontent.com/pod-product-compliance
Lightning Source LLC
Chambersburg PA
CBHW070644290526
45790CB00001B/185